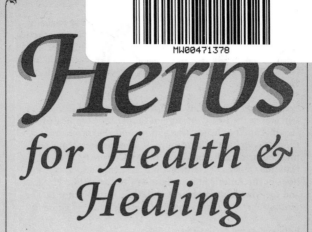

Herbs

for Health &
Healing

Jill Stansbury, N.D.

Consultant: Paul Bergner

Publications International, Ltd.

Dr. Jill E. Stansbury is a naturopathic physician specializing in botanical medicine. Stansbury maintains a private practice in Washington and is chair of the Botanical Medicine Department at National College of Naturopathic Medicine in Portland, Oregon. She is a contributing editor for *Medical Herbalism*.

Paul Bergner is editor of *Medical Herbalism* and Clinic Director at the Rocky Mountain Center for Botanical Studies. He edits and publishes *The Naturopathic Physician* and *Clinical Nutrition Update* journals. Bergner frequently lectures on medical herbalism at Bastyr University, at the National College of Naturopathic Medicine, and at conventions of the American Association of Naturopathic Physicians and the American Herbalists Guild. He is the author of *The Healing Power of Garlic* and *The Healing Power of Ginseng*.

Editorial Assistance: Jeffrey Laign
Illustrations: Virge Kask, Bev Benner, Marlene Hill-Donnelly, Susan Spellman

Cover photo credit: Spencer Jones/FPG International.
Inside photo credit: Courtesy of the Lloyd Library and Museum, Cincinnati, Ohio.

CONTENTS

❧

INTRODUCTION

❧

*H*ERBS HAVE LONG INTRIGUED US—and for good reason. Because of their potential as food and as medicine, they have enjoyed a special relationship with humans throughout the ages.

To our ancestors, knowledge of herbs meant survival. But the passage of time did not diminish human beings' respect for the herb. Druids revered the oak and mistletoe, both rich in medicinal attributes. In the Eastern world, physicians wrote tomes on herbal remedies, some prized to this day as authoritative medical sources. Later, the Greeks and Romans cultivated herbs for medicinal as well as culinary uses. Hippocrates, considered the father of Western medicine, prescribed scores of curative herbs and taught his students how to use them. The search for precious herbs and spices led Europeans to the New World. There they found scores of new plants which they brought back with them to the courts of England, Spain, and France.

The development of pharmaceutical drugs some 100 years ago changed our focus from herbs and natural healing to the new "wonder drugs." Medical practice turned away from botanicals and embraced these new chemical-based medicines. In addition, the Industrial Revolution meant urbanization, and city dwellers, who now had limited access to gardens, welcomed the convenience of shopping for—instead of growing—their medicines and foods.

In recent years, however, herbs have enjoyed a renaissance. Though lifesavers in countless cases, pharmaceutical drugs proved not to be the magic bullets we'd hoped for. Seeking ways to feel better without the side effects of pharmaceutical drugs, countless people are rediscovering herbs as natural remedies.

What exactly is an herb? No group of plants is more difficult to define. In general, an herb is a seed-producing plant that dies down at the end of the growing season and is noted for its aromatic and/or medicinal qualities. (Chapter 2 explains how to select herbs based on these qualities.) Among the most utilitarian of plants, herbs lend themselves to a seemingly endless array of medicinal preparations. And you don't have to be a pharmacist—or a shaman—to make them. You just have to read Chapter 3, "Preparing Herbal Medicines." The remainder of the book focuses on the use of these amazing plants to heal.

Like other healing traditions, herbal medicine recognizes and respects the forces of nature: Health is seen as the proper balance or rhythm of natural forces while disease is an imbalance of these forces. Because the forces of nature are not easily grasped and manipulated, herbal traditions turn to the earth's masters of natural balance and symmetry—plants.

Indeed, plants are ideal biochemical medicines. We have built-in systems for metabolizing plants and using their energies. But our bodies have difficulty metabolizing and excreting synthetic chemical medicines. And think about the negative terms used to describe the actions of synthetic pharmaceuticals: they suppress, they fight, they inhibit. They do little to support overall health. Medicines made from plants, on the other hand, tend to nourish the body without taxing it, to support the body system rather than suppressing it.

Some pharmacists and pharmacologists argue that synthetic drugs derived from plants have an action identical to the active constituents in the plants. (Constituents are the elements of the plant; active constituents are the elements that produce an effect.) While this is true in some cases (digoxin and ephedrine, to name just two), most synthetic drugs are not identical to their natural counterparts.

Most plants contain a dozen or more different constituents. The idea that we can entirely duplicate the action of a plant by simply synthesizing a single active constituent is somewhat misguided. Part of a plant's healing effect is due to the sum total of all the constituents. To isolate certain constituents is to rob a plant of its deeper healing potential. This concept of a healing vitality or life force in the whole plant is central to the tradition of herbal medicine and is recognized in all the ancient medical systems.

There's no doubt that pharmaceuticals have their place. They enable dramatic alterations of biochemical processes—they can halt severe inflammation, slow the rate of the heart or respiration, or stimulate the bowels to move. These medicines are often necessary in emergencies, acute conditions, and cases of severe illness.

But plants offer us nourishment and healing actions that synthetic medications cannot. Many herbs have shown profound healing effects when used as tonics over long periods. Furthermore, synthetic drugs are combined with waxes, stabilizers, tableting agents, and coatings. Plants, on the other hand, are complex collections of naturally occurring and nourishing substances that may have vital roles in health, including vitamins, minerals, amino acids, fatty acids, fiber, and bioflavonoids. Synthetic drugs can also cause side effects and long-term toxicities that are rare in plants. Botanical medications restore the body's processes to normal function; synthetic drugs can push these processes to unnecessary extremes.

Use this book to explore the healing potential of herbs. Whether you make your own medicines or purchase herbal preparations, we believe you, too, will experience the benefits of herbal medicine. Here's to your health—your natural health.

HERBAL MEDICINE
YESTERDAY AND TODAY

❧

*I*T WAS OUR ANCESTORS, in their search for nourishment, who uncovered the roots of medicine. The Neanderthal and Paleolithic peoples
were hunters and gatherers who lived intimately
with nature, using plants as food, clothing, shelter,
tools, weapons, and medicine. They discovered
certain plants could optimize their health while
others reduced fertility or made them ill. As they
learned which plants were not poisonous, which
were nourishing, and which were palatable, they
also noted which could calm a nauseous stomach,
ease the pains of childbirth, and heal wounds.
Some Stone Age artifacts appear to be tools that
could grind grains, roots, seeds, and bark—pre-
cursors of the mortar and pestle we use today.

ANCIENT INDIA AND
AYURVEDIC MEDICINE
(ABOUT 10,000 B.C. TO PRESENT)

Some of the oldest known writings are clay tablets
unearthed in what is now the Middle East. Many
of these ancient clay tablets mention healing
plants. Within these early writings are four books
of classic wisdom, called the Vedas, from which
the system of Ayurvedic medicine, as well as the
Hindu religion, arose. Believed to have been
recanted orally since at least 10,000 B.C., the information within the Rig Veda—the oldest of the

four books—describes this
ancient medical system.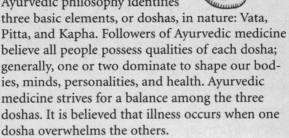

Ayurveda means science of life.
Deeply respectful of nature,
Ayurvedic philosophy identifies
three basic elements, or doshas, in nature: Vata,
Pitta, and Kapha. Followers of Ayurvedic medicine
believe all people possess qualities of each dosha;
generally, one or two dominate to shape our bodies, minds, personalities, and health. Ayurvedic
medicine strives for a balance among the three
doshas. It is believed that illness occurs when one
dosha overwhelms the others.

Ayurvedic medicine looks to nature as the source
of wellness, thus its use of healing plants. An
Ayurvedic doctor or herbalist begins by identify-
ing which dosha type(s) an individual is; this
allows him or her to use an herb with a corre-
sponding physiologic action. A person who tends
to have dominant Vata energies, for example, will
benefit from plants that decrease excess Vata
and/or increase Kapha and Pitta. The effective use
of herbs in Ayurvedic medicine requires an inti-
mate understanding of the natural forces within a
plant.

ANCIENT CHINA AND TAOISM
(5000 B.C. TO PRESENT)

Ancient Asian cultures also embraced the idea that
one should seek a balance with the natural forces
within all life forms. Chinese Toaism embraces a

bipolar medical system rather than the tripolar system of the Ayurvedic doshas. The life force is seen as the ever-churning circular motion of two opposing actions, yin and yang. All diseases are understood as an imbalance of yin and yang. The Chinese believe that qi (pronounced chee and sometimes written as chi), or vital energy, is responsible for health, and an imbalance of qi results in illness.

All matter, including plants and animals, is yin and yang (although one usually dominates); therefore, plant qi can be used to balance animal qi. A disturbance in a person's qi may affect the balance of yin and yang. For example, if qi is blocked, yang may predominate. Some herbs are predominantly yin tonics, some are yang tonics, and most are a complex combination of yin and yang. Chinese herbalists must be familiar with each plant's energy to prescribe the herbal remedies with the most healing potential.

Ancient Chinese healers were quite sophisticated in their use of plant medicines. One surviving materia medica (Latin for "on medicine"; the term refers to a list of medicinal substances) of more than 365 plants is the *Pen-ts'ao Ching (The Classic of Herbs)*. This oldest-known Chinese pharmacopoeia is said to be the work of the Emperor Shen Nung who ruled in the 28th century B.C. The *Pen-ts'ao Ching* lists plants still in use today, including ma huang, ginger, and cinnamon.

Other written records of Chinese herbalism include the *Huang ti Nei Ching*, written in 2500 B.C. by Huang ti, the "Yellow Emperor." The *Nei Ching*, as it was later known, is a comprehensive review of Chinese medical arts. A classic on internal medicine, it is still used today in acupuncture schools in the United States. The *Li Shih-Chen* is another ancient Chinese herbal materia medica written by a Chinese scholar by the same name. It was translated into English and published in Britain in 1596 after centuries of use in China. This compendium, which lists more than 2,000 drugs and 8,000 prescriptions, is still studied by traditional Chinese physicians.

ANCIENT EGYPT
(4000 B.C. TO 1000 B.C.)

The Eber's papyrus is one of Egypt's most important surviving medical writings. Dating from approximately 1550 B.C., this 65-foot papyrus scroll was discovered in 1873 by Georg Ebers, a German Egyptologist. The document includes both herbal and medical therapies, including numerous substances still thought to be medicinally active, such as garlic and moldy bread. The Egyptians had a sophisticated knowledge of plants, as their practice of using myrrh in embalming attests.

ANCIENT GREECE
(1000 B.C. TO A.D. 1)

In Greek mythology Asclepias, the Greek god of healing and medicine, carried a caduceus. In ancient Greece, the caduceus, a snake wrapped around the staff of knowledge, symbolized knowledge and healing. Today, the caduceus remains the symbol of medical science.

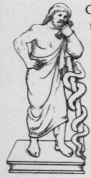

Greek healers and physicians came to be known as Asclepiads. Aristotle, who lived approximately 384–322 B.C., was believed to be a descendant of Asclepias. Perhaps best known for his school of philosophy, founded about 335 B.C., Aristotle also wrote hundreds of books on numerous subjects, including one work that described 500 plants, called *De Plants*.

The Iron Age witnessed the flourishing of civilizations. During that time, the first medical schools were formed, foreign lands were explored, and goods were traded. The spice trade was particularly strong; ultimately, it stimulated transoceanic explorations by the Europeans. Many kings and emperors hoped to lay claim to new lands and the resources these lands offered. Poisons were frequently used to deal with enemies and achieve these goals.

One of the medical schools founded in Alexandria emphasized the study of poisonous plants. Crateuas, who lived about 100 B.C., was a plant collector and herbalist for King Mithradates VI, known as The King of Poisons. (Mithradates is said to have taken various poisons prepared by Crateuas, increasing the doses over time so his body would develop a tolerance for them. He hoped to make himself immune to the threat of poisoning.) The drawings by Crateuas are the earliest known botanical illustrations. His was the first illustrated pharmacopoeia, which classified the plants and explained their medicinal uses.

Pendanius Dioscorides, a Greek who lived around A.D. 100, served as a physician to the Roman army. He traveled extensively throughout Europe and published the five books commonly referred to as *De Materia Medica*. A compendium of nearly 600 plants, it was the leading pharmacologic text for 16 centuries. This thorough work included most of the previously existing herbal literature.

A review of classical Greek medicine would not be complete without mention of Hippocrates. Born about 460 B.C., Hippocrates was the son of the Asclepiad physician Heraklides, but he eschewed the Asclepiads for their many superstitious practices. Considered the Father of Medicine, Hippocrates believed in gathering data and employing observation and experiments in his practice and study of medicine. (He helped commence the Age of Reason.) Hippocrates banished magic, superstition, and incantations. Instead, he embraced the life force, the laws of nature, the body's innate ability to heal itself, and the healing 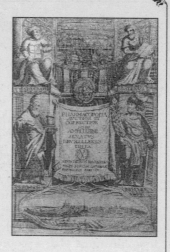 power of nature—all principles that relate to herbalism. He stated, "Nature heals, the physician is only Nature's assistant." Out of the school of medicine named after Hippocrates came the Hippocratic Oath, a code of medical ethics taken by physicians, which remains in use today.

Galen was a Roman physician during the period that Rome was the hub of the world (around A.D. 130–200). As a result of his thorough medical research on cadavers, he is sometimes referred to as the Father of Anatomy. (During the era of gladiators, vicious battles were common, and Galen gained some of his knowledge of anatomy by attending to injured warriors.) Galen authored an astounding 400 books, half of them on medical subjects, including *De Simplicus,* an herbal. He created potent medicines by combining plant, animal, and mineral substances. One well-known recipe, Galen's Theriac, had an opium base and more than 70 ingredients, including animal flesh, herbs, minerals, honey, and wine. It remained in use for several centuries.

ARABIA
(A.D. 800 TO PRESENT)

Arabic medicine was derived from classical Greek medicine—its name, Unani Tibb, means Greek medicine. The Arabian physician Avicenna is credited as the first to distill essential oils from aromatic plants. One of his books, the five-volume *Canon of Medicine,* an authoritative and monumental compendium of all medical knowledge at the time, remained in use in Europe for more than 700 years from its publication about A.D. 1020. Unani Tibb remains the primary medical system for about 200 million people in the Middle East and southern Asia.

EUROPE IN THE ELIZABETHAN ERA
(LATE 1500S TO EARLY 1600S)

The Swiss physician Paracelsus lived from 1493 to 1541. Paracelsus traveled throughout Europe studying chemistry, alchemy, and metallurgy and their application to medicine. He reasoned that plants had some sort of active chemicals that were responsible for their actions. Because Paracelsus wrote in the common language of the people rather than in Latin, he was lauded by folk healers, and, likewise, Paracelsus respected them. He

believed these healers possessed ancient knowledge passed down from the ancient Magi. The
Magi were adept at using belladonna (atropine),
mandragora (mandrake), and papaver (opium
poppy) as anesthetics. Perhaps Paracelsus's study
of the Magi led to his thoughts on homeopathy
(the use of extreme dilutions of plant, animal, and
mineral products to promote healing), which
closely approximate modern homeopathic philosophy.

An English apothecary, Nicolas Culpeper
sought to remove power from
medical doctors and put it in
the hands of the apothecary
profession. He supported
educating people to care for
themselves—especially those who could not afford
doctor visits. He disturbed the entire medical profession by translating the *London Pharmacopoeia*
from Latin to English in 1649, putting it in the
hands of the common people. Culpeper is also
known for his association with the Doctrine of
Signatures, an ancient concept that held that the
physiologic action of a particular plant on the
human body can be learned or inferred from
observing the plant and getting to know its char-
acter and appearance.

John Gerard, an Englishman who lived around the
same time as Culpeper, was a barber-surgeon. In
those days, many physicians dispensed medicine
only. Barber-surgeons filled the gap by offering

minor surgical procedures. The red and blue striped barber pole is a remnant of the old symbol used by the barber-surgeons—the blue stripe represents venous blood and the red stripe represents arterial blood. And yes, you could also get your hair cut while you were undergoing surgery. Gerard published the *General History of Plants,* more commonly known as *Gerard's Herbal,* in 1597.

EARLY AMERICAN MEDICINE

The medicine of early Americans was a blend of Native American remedies and numerous European traditions. The early settlers brought seeds and plants with them from Europe to the new land; some native American plants, such as plantain, dandelion, and red clover, were already familiar to them. Many households had a family herbal—held in nearly equal esteem with the family Bible—to which they often referred during times of illness. As the colonies grew, the new Americans learned from each other and the Native Americans, incorporating the practices of the different cultures into their medical knowledge. This broad knowledge base gave rise to the early American Eclectic physicians.

The Eclectics, whose philosophy was popular from the end of the 1800s through the early 1900s, were licensed physicians, but they opposed some of the current medical trends such as bloodletting and the use of arsenic as a medicine. The Eclectics espoused tailoring the medicine very closely to each individual and defined very specifically the herbs that best treated a particular condition. The temperature of the patient; the appearance of the skin, tongue, and eyes; the gait; and the pulse were all carefully noted. Their skill in noting which plant was most specific for which symptom or collection of symptoms made their system of prescribing known as "specific medication."

MODERN TIMES

Herbal medicine and other alternative therapies, such as homeopathy and hydrotherapy, flourished in early America. In fact, at the beginning of the 20th century, 25 percent of all doctors practiced some form of homeopathy, and a homeopath could be found on the staff of nearly every major hospital. So prominent and popular, in fact, were all types of healing arts that there is reported to have been a glut of doctors—all types of physicians competed for business.

The American Medical Association (AMA) was formed in the 1840s at a time when allopathic (conventional, Western) medicine was in decline, and homeopathy and herbal medicine were the dominant medical systems. The decline of traditional allopathic medicine followed the success of the homeopaths and herbal physicians in treating people during epidemic diseases in the cities in the 1830s—diseases the allopathic physicians were not equipped to handle. The AMA was organized to protect the interests of this declining profession; the organization chose its weapons of protection well.

In 1910, the Carnegie Foundation for the Advancement of Teaching published a report by educator Abraham Flexner. The Flexner Report examined American medical schools and education programs and recommended approval only to allopathic-oriented schools. Foundation grants and state regulators, in general, followed the Flexner Report's recommendations, with prompting by the emerging drug companies and the political lobbying of the AMA. This economic and political trend effectively killed the Eclectic and homeopathic medical professions, which formerly had been on an equal footing with the allopaths. It also eliminated the semi-professional herbalists. Formal medical-level herbalism was kept alive into the 1930s by a few remaining Eclectic physicians as well as by an emerging naturopathic medical profession.

When pharmaceutical science emerged around the early 1900s, the allopathic practitioners in the United States relied solely on pharmaceuticals at the expense of herbal medicines. Penicillin and other drugs saved millions of lives; indeed, it seemed that pharmaceuticals were long-awaited miracles.

But pharmaceuticals cannot nourish or strengthen the health and vitality of the entire body. They usually address only a single symptom and force certain pharmacologic effects. Many pharmaceuticals achieve these effects at a cost, which we refer to as side effects. For example, while antibiotics kill bacteria, they don't address the underlying cause of infection. And at the same time they kill harmful bacteria, they also destroy beneficial bacteria (such as *Lactobacillus acidophilus*) within the intestines and vagina, making it easier for yeast and other pathogens to move in. More troubling is that many types of infection are becoming resistant to pharmaceuticals. Widespread use of antibiotics in medicines—as well as their use in animals whose meat is intended for human consumption—may be responsible for the evolution of super bacteria that are resistant to most pharmaceuticals.

Armed with the realization that pharmaceuticals are not the panacea once imagined, many people are returning to natural therapies. Herbalism in the United States has been undergoing a renaissance since the early 1970s, with the reemergence of the naturopathic medical profession after its decline in the 1950s and 1960s. In the last ten years, at least six schools of herbal medicine have emerged in North America, now graduating several hundred clinically trained herbalists a year. Research dollars are increasingly becoming available to investigate botanical therapies. Nurseries stock a wide assortment of culinary and medicinal herbs. Public seminars and symposia on herbal medicine are often filled to capacity. Numerous books, journals, and community programs have emerged to help the public gain a working knowledge of this important field of medicine.

A GUIDE TO SHOPPING FOR HERBS

❧

*T*HE RECENT INTEREST IN HERBS and herbal medicines has led to a boom in herbal products. A whole gamut of herb types and strengths is now available, and there's a variety of ways to use and consume them. With so many herb products available, you may not know where to start. But don't despair: Anyone can learn how to use the most common herbs—safely and easily.

You can purchase herbal medicines at your local health food store or natural-product pharmacy. You can also make herbal remedies yourself, which is a less expensive—and more satisfying—alternative. Whichever route you choose to take, you need to know a few herb basics before you head to the store.

PURCHASING HERBS TO MAKE YOUR OWN PREPARATIONS

When buying a bulk herb for use as a cooking spice or tea, or for making your own homemade herbal products, choose herbs with a strong aroma, color, and flavor. Selection is fairly easy once you become familiar with an herb's characteristic odor, taste, and appearance. Many grocery stores carry fresh culinary herbs in the produce department, and health food stores and specialty herb stores carry dried herbs in bulk bins or jars.

Compare an herb's character-
istics in preparations, too.
If an herbal tea imparts a
strong color to the water,
with a good aroma and
strong flavor, its quality is
probably good. Teas and
tinctures with pale colors
and weak flavors are of
poor quality. If possible,
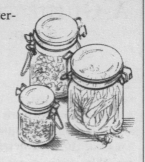
select teas that have been harvested less than one
year ago. Look for tinctures made from fresh
plants.

You will most likely want to start with the inexpensive, grow-your-own or readily available herbs.
Be sure to begin with herbs considered entirely
nontoxic. Be aware, however, that "safe" and "nontoxic" do not mean 100 percent reaction-free; they
do mean nonlethal and almost always harmless.

Individual reactions can occur from any substance,
including mint, garlic, or alfalfa. Always use caution when using an herbal medicine for the first
time—don't take handfuls of capsules or drink
pots of tea. Begin with 2 to 3 capsules or 1 to 2
cups of tea daily for a few days to see how your
body reacts. People who have a history of reacting
to prescription drugs or people who are very sensitive to perfumes or soaps should be cautious.
For any serious or persistent health complaints,
you should consult a naturopathic or other type
of physician.

Herbal teas and essential oils from an herbalist are likely to be much stronger than their grocery store counterparts. Even common spices an herbalist dispenses, such as cinnamon or ginger, are likely to be of stronger color, flavor, and smell than the cinnamon or ginger in your spice rack. But as interest in herbs grows, fresh herbs and specialty teas of good, strong quality are becoming more accessible to the general consumer.

In general, an herb's potency as a flavoring is intimately linked to its potency as a medicine, and the two actions are likely to diminish equally with time. This is because much of an herb's medicinal actions are due to essential (volatile) oils—the oils in herbs we cherish as aromatic and flavoring substances. As the name "volatile" suggests, these are fairly unstable compounds; they are one of the first constituents in any herb to decompose and become less potent. So if an herb or spice has a strong smell and flavor, it is probably still strong as a medicine. As the flavor and aroma wane, the medicinal activity wanes concurrently.

Dried and powdered herbs remain at full potency for about a year. Most tinctures and essential oils maintain a good, strong potency for three to five years.

PURCHASING HERBAL PREPARATIONS

When buying herbs in capsule or tablet form, it's often impossible to assess the quality of the herbs. Naturopathic physicians, herbalists, or individuals who have used the product are good sources of information. It's a good idea to do some careful study about the herbs you are considering. Make sure they are indicated for the condition you wish to treat or prevent, and make sure you understand the appropriate therapeutic dosage.

Increasingly, herb suppliers are "standardizing" the botanical extracts they sell to consumers. This means these herbal preparations have been tested to determine the type and amount of at least one chemical constituent contained in the plant. Standardization sounds like a good idea. But the practice has its pros and cons.

The good news is that standardization ensures the potency of an herbal product. Many of the healing properties of ginkgo, for example, are thought to reside in chemicals called heterosides. Thus, if you buy a standardized ginkgo preparation, you can be fairly certain you're getting a sufficient amount of heterosides. The problem is, ginkgo also contains flavonoids and super oxide dismutase. Should we standardize for these chemicals? If we discover five more active constituents in the next decade, will they all need to be standardized? If so, we can expect to be paying plenty for the herbs we buy.

Another problem with standardization is that as we study the medicinal effects of herbs, we're learning that healing may result not from a single element contained in a plant, but from a complex combination of constituents. Standardization implies that an herb is good only for the standardized constituent. But herbs contain many nourishing substances, and, unlike drugs, herbs are not administered to produce a single chemical effect. If we begin to value plants for their standardized chemicals only, it won't be long before pharmaceutical companies are isolating extracts and packaging them as drugs. And that's not what herbal medicine is about.

Herbal healing is a holistic process. Forgoing traditional Western thinking, herbalists do not use drugs to suppress symptoms of an illness. Herbs are meant to spur our bodies to heal naturally. So next time you get a headache, cold, or minor cut or scrape, pay a visit to nature's pharmacy. Of course, you should never attempt to diagnose a serious illness and treat it yourself. In such cases, seek advice from a physician.

PURCHASING AND USING ESSENTIAL OILS

Essential, or volatile, oils are aromatic, fragrant substances in plants. Essential oils enhance the aroma and flavor of foods and beverages and pro-

RESPECT MOTHER NATURE

If you are interested in herbs and natural medicine, it's likely you are also interested in nature. Another responsibility you have as an herb consumer is to investigate, when possible, the ethical practices of the supplier. Were the plants cultivated, or were they taken from the wild, a process called "wildcrafting"? If wildcrafted, is the plant plentiful, or is it a rare plant that may be further disrupted by harvesting? Was care taken to avoid harvesting from roadways, under power lines, or near toxic waters or environments? If cultivated, was the plant grown organically? If not, what pesticide or other residues might be in the plant? When was the plant harvested, and how was it processed? Does the grower or harvester process the plant, or was it shipped somewhere else for processing? Sadly, even some of the firms that sell their products widely in health food stores use half-truths in their marketing and in their claims of product integrity. An herbalist can help you identify the ethical firms.

vide scent to potpourri and perfumes. You can also use them in herbal medicines; the smell of essential oils alone is thought to have medicinal value.

Aromatherapy is the practice of using fragrant plants as medicine. Different natural aromas have different effects on our physiology and, particularly, our emotional state. Inhaling various aromas can promote relaxation, increase mental awareness, or improve sleep, for example.

Many health food, nutrition, and specialty stores carry essential oils in small glass bottles at a reasonable price. Many of the oils such as peppermint, orange, or cinnamon are quite inexpensive; you'll pay more for precious flower oils such as rose and jasmine. But because you use essential oils in very tiny quantities, your initial investment is likely to last many years.

Be aware that "perfume" oils are not the same as essential oils. Essential oils are natural plant constituents that have been extracted from the plant. They are oily liquids. Perfume oils are synthetic and are not derived from plants.

You can use essential oils medicinally in a variety of ways. Essential oils are typically dispensed by placing a small amount of the oil into another liquid. An essential oil such as eucalyptus added to a pot of steaming water becomes a natural vaporizer for a stuffy nose, sinus infection, or chest cold. Applied topically in a liniment or massage oil, essential oils can treat sore muscles, infections, and inflammation.

The use of essential oils topically requires great care: Many essential oils such as thyme, peppermint, and cinnamon can irritate and even burn the skin. While other essential oils such as tea tree and lavender tend to be less irritating, as a general rule, always dilute essential oils with almond oil or a vegetable oil such as olive oil, and use them cautiously on the skin. Be extra careful when using essential oils with children, highly allergic individuals, and those with sensitive skin. Do not use them on pets.

To achieve the effects of aromatherapy, you can add essential oils to potpourri or place a few drops on a cotton ball and tuck it into your pillow or in a dresser drawer. You can also add essential oils to the rinse cycle of your washing machine. You can wear essential oils like perfumes (diluted, of course!), or place a few drops on a light ring or special aromatherapy diffuser that disperses the aroma without heat. Rubbed into the temples or brushed through the hair, essential oils can relieve headaches; added to bath water, they can promote relaxation.

CONSULTING AN HERBALIST

You can find an herbalist by checking with the American Herbalist Guild or with the American Association of Naturopathic Physicians listed in the Resources section, pages 239–240. An herbalist or naturopathic physician will want to know all the details about your complaint—how long you've had it, what makes it better or worse, what other complaints might accompany it. Is there an emotional component? Does it interfere with your sleep? Does it change with your diet, the season, your menstrual cycle, the amount of stress you're under? An herbalist will also want to know about your entire state of health, including your medical history—are you healthy otherwise, or do you have other complaints? What do you typically eat and drink? Do you exercise regularly? How do you relax?

In addition to performing a regular physical examination, a naturopathic physician will note the quality of your pulse, the look of your eyes, the glow of your skin, and your general vitality. An herbalist will likely note if you appear tense or sluggish, if you are hot or cold, animated or withdrawn, sharp and alert or dull and out of touch. After spending some time getting to know you, an herbalist can generally make very specific and fine-tuned recommendations.

THE REGULATION AND SAFETY OF HERBAL MEDICINES

The U.S. Food and Drug Administration (FDA) regulates food and drugs, but, at the present time, no agency regulates herbs. To be regulated by the FDA, herbs would have to be declared either a food or drug.

Some of the current disorganization revolves around the difficulty of fitting herbs into these pigeonholes. Herbs are very nourishing and contain vitamins and minerals, so they could be classified as foods. But herbs also contain pharmacologically active substances, some of them quite strong in their action, so they could also be considered drugs. And some herbs such as nettles,

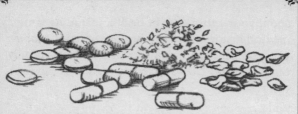

spirulina, and alfalfa are more like foods, while other herbs such as ma huang and kava kava are more like drugs. Coffee certainly has a druglike action, but it is regulated as a food and not a drug. A food does not require extensive testing for the FDA to allow its consumption in the United States. A drug, however, requires extensive testing before the FDA has enough information to allow its use in the United States. If claims are made, for example, that an herb can help control blood sugar, it must be considered a drug. The question that follows is, does this drug need FDA approval? Or, like foods, if the herb-drug has a substantial history of safe use, can its approval be based on historical rather than empirical evidence?

The process of gathering data and empirical evidence for drug approval typically takes many millions of dollars. Large pharmaceutical companies have enormous research budgets to run theoretical studies, animal studies, and, finally, human clinical trials of a drug to get it approved. Pharmaceutical companies are willing to spend large sums of money to ensure a drug's approval because they will earn billions of dollars from sales of the approved drug. Herb growers, processors, and distributors, however, do not typically have million-dollar research departments; even if they did, it isn't worthwhile to spend millions proving the efficacy of an herb that consumers could grow in their backyards. Pharmaceutical companies are entitled to patent their approved drug. Herbs are not patentable, so a company that funded research could not expect exclusive rights to that herb, and even the knowledge acquired through research would soon become public domain.

This is the root of the dilemma surrounding the regulation of botanical medicines. Perhaps a separate regulatory agency for herbs will emerge. Perhaps the FDA will begin to study the vast history of use of many botanicals and officially approve some of them without million-dollar clinical testing. Until that time, the consumer must bear the burden of responsibility for use of herbal medicines.

When using any herbal remedy, educate yourself about the herbs you're interested in. Do not take any substance unless it is indicated for the problem you have. Do not assume an herb is safe because it's available in a health food store. Though most products are safe, some may have been formulated with only a rudimentary knowledge of herbs and could prove harmful. Consult a physician or herbalist if you have any questions about the herbs you wish to use or the condition you wish to treat.

PREPARING HERBAL MEDICINES AT HOME

❧

*A*NCIENT CULTURES REGARDED the harvest season as a sacred time—a time to reap the fruits of a year's hard labor and rejoice in the abundance of the earth. Harvest your herbs with no less reverence. In fact, the connection with nature may play a role in maintaining your health. Clearly, spending time in a forest or meadow feels very different from spending time in an office or factory or an urban setting. Handling herbs and handcrafting them into medicines is a healing activity in itself!

GATHERING HERBS

Gathering plants you've grown yourself gives you a tremendous sense of accomplishment, but you may also collect herbs growing wild. Gathering herbs from the wild is referred to as "wildcrafting." If you pick wild herbs, however, be certain you've identified them properly. Some poisonous herbs resemble harmless ones. Also, make sure the area where you're wildcrafting is free of pesticides, chemical sprays, or other pollutants. Avoid picking herbs growing along busy roads or highways where car exhaust can contaminate them.

Do not harvest rare or endangered plants from the wild. Many plant species are threatened through both overharvesting and loss of habitat. Echinacea, ginseng, and goldenseal species, for example, are all declining. Certainly we still have some dandelion and red clover to spare, but cultivating herbs yourself can help preserve the native habitats of some endangered plant species.

HARVESTING YOUR HERBS

As a general rule, harvest the leaves of an herb when the plant is about to flower—usually in the spring or fall. (Plants are very high in volatile oils right before they flower.) Harvest roots and bark in the fall and winter months when the plant is dormant and its nutrients are in storage.

Gather herbs in the morning on a dry day. Herbs that are dry when harvested are less likely to mold or spoil during processing. Avoid washing leaves and flowers of herbs after you've harvested them. If the herbs are covered with dirt or dust, rinse them off with a garden hose or watering can, then allow the herbs to dry for a day or two before picking them. When wildcrafting, shake the water off wet herbs; you may also try drying wild herbs by gently blotting them with a towel. The root of the herb is the only part of that plant you should wash thoroughly after harvesting.

Harvesting the seeds of an herb requires a little more intuition. You need to check your plants everyday, and be prepared to harvest the seeds as soon as you notice they've begun to dry. (Timing is crucial: You must allow the seeds to ripen, but catch them before they fall off the plant.) Carefully snap off seed heads over a large paper bag, allowing the seeds to fall into it. Leave the seeds in the bag until they have dried completely.

DRYING HERBS

Herbal preparations often require the use of dried herbs. To dry herbs, hang them upside down until they are crisp. If you have a spare countertop or closet shelf, you can spread the herbs over newspaper or paper towels. (Keep the herbs evenly distributed, avoiding thick, wet piles.) Cover the herbs with a paper towel or a very thin piece of cheesecloth to prevent dust from settling.

Do not dry herbs in direct sunlight. Dry herbs in an area that is hot, well ventilated, and free of moisture, such as a barn, loft, breezeway, or covered porch. In these conditions, the moisture will evaporate quickly from the plants, but the aromatic oils will remain in the leaves.

You can also use a food dehydrator (use the lowest setting) to dry your herbs. If you're handy with a saw and hammer and nails, you can build a drying cabinet in which the herbs sit on screens and warm air circulates through the screens. A drying

DRYING METHODS

Method 1: Use a rubber band to bind herb and flower branches. Hang them upside down in a hot, dry place that receives little or no light. Ensure that your drying area has good air circulation to prevent mold from developing on the plants. Keep herb bunches small if your drying area is humid.

Method 2: Remove petals from flowers and leaves from stems and spread them evenly on a clean window screen. Leave space between herb pieces to ensure adequate air circulation. Place the screen out of the wind in a hot, dry place that receives little light.

Method 3: To dry seeds, hang bundles of plants as in Method 1, placing each bundle inside a large brown paper bag to catch the seeds. Or hang bunches from poles laid across an open cardboard box lined with a sheet of paper.

Method 4: Before drying roots, scrub them thoroughly. Split thick roots lengthwise. Slice roots in ¼-inch-thick pieces. Air dry as in Method 2, or spread roots on cookie sheets and dry them in a conventional oven at the lowest setting.

Hint: You can dry more than just herbs! Dried apple and pear peels add taste to teas. Use dried orange, lemon, and other citrus rinds in teas, potpourri, and herbal bath blends. Dried blueberry and strawberry leaves add nutrients and color to winter teas. Use a dehydrator to dry mashed, over-ripe fruit; break the fruit rolls apart and add to teas and dessert sauces.

cabinet can be a plain cupboard in a warm, dry location, or it can be a fancy version with a solar or electric heater with fans to circulate the air. Whatever drying method you use, the optimal temperature for drying herbs is approximately 85 degrees Fahrenheit. Higher temperatures can harm the herbs and dissipate the volatile oils.

It may take up to a week to dry some herbs, depending on the thickness of the plant's leaves and stem. As soon as leaves are fully dry—but before they become brittle—strip them from the stems. Store the leaves immediately in airtight containers to preserve their flavor and aroma. Label the containers with the herb name and date stored.

STORING HERBS

Once you've fully dried your herbs, don't delay in storing them in airtight containers or your herbs will lose essential oils, the source of an herb's flavor and perfume. Simply crumble the herbs before storing. Avoid grinding and powdering herbs because they won't retain their flavor as long.

Glass jars with tight-sealing lids or glass stoppers are ideal for storing dried herbs. You may also use porcelain canisters that close tightly, plastic pill holders with tight covers, and sealable plastic bags, buckets, or barrels for large herb pieces.

Storing Herbs

Follow these steps to store herbs:

1. You can store herbs in sealable jars, canisters, pill bottles, and plastic bags. Thoroughly wash, rinse, and dry containers and lids to rid them of previous lingering odors.

2. When herbs are dry—but before they crumble when touched—remove their leaves, flowers, or seeds and put them in a bowl. Leave these pieces whole or crumble them with your fingers or a mortar and pestle. Note: Herbs that are ground or powdered don't retain their flavor as long.

3. Using a clean sheet of paper rolled into a funnel, pour the herbs into dry containers.

4. Label containers clearly with the name of the herb and its year of harvest. (Without labels you'll soon find it difficult to keep your inventories straight.)

5. Store herbs in a dark place to preserve their colors and flavors. If no such space is available, be sure to use tinted nonmetallic containers with tight covers or tinted sealable jars.

Store herbs in a dark place to preserve their color and flavor. If you must store herbs in a lighted area, keep them in dark-colored jars that block out most of the light. The worst place to keep herbs is in a spice rack over the stove: Heat from cooking will cause your herbs to lose their flavor quickly. Remember to label each container, including its contents and date of harvest.

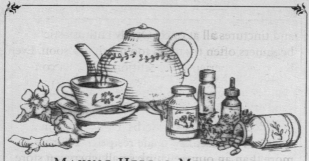

Making Herbal Medicines

You've grown your herbs, gathered them, and
dried them. The next step is to prepare them.
Preparing herbs is simple and easy—not to mention economical.

The goal of the herbalist is to release the volatile
oils, antibiotics, aromatics, and other healing
chemicals an herb contains. You can use dried,
powdered herbs to make pills, capsules, and
lozenges or add herbs to water to brew infusions,
better known as teas. You can soak herbs in alcohol to produce long-lasting tinctures. A spoonful
(or more) of sweetener helps the medicine go
down in the form of delectable syrups, jellies, and
conserves. You can mash herbs for poultices and
plasters. Or you can harness the powers of herbs
by adding them to oils to make salves, liniments,
and creams.

First Steps

Lay out all the cooking, storage, and labeling
materials you'll need to prepare your herbal home
remedies. Don't attempt to make salves, syrups,

and tinctures all at once. Overly enthusiastic beginners often try to do too much too soon. Even the most experienced practitioner can get confused and make mistakes. Concentrate on making only one type of herbal remedy at a time.

Don't overharvest your herbs. Don't bring in a basketful of rosemary if the recipe calls for no more than an ounce. Think small when you store your herbs, too. Salves and other preparations tend to last longer when stored in small batches. If you intend to save these medicines for longer than a few months, tightly stopper bottles, seal jars with wax, and refrigerate liquid preparations.

Using the basic recipes described in this chapter, you can create your own versions of such delightful herbal preparations as tummy-calming teas, snappy vinegars, sensuous massage oils, and body-smoothing creams.

TEAS

One of the easiest and most popular ways of preparing an herbal medicine is to brew a tea. There are two types of teas: infusions and decoctions. If you have ever poured hot water over a tea bag, you have made an infusion; an infusion is herbs steeped in water. A decoction is herbs boiled in water. When you simmer cinnamon sticks and cloves in apple cider, you're making a decoction.

In general, delicate leaves and flowers are best infused; boiling may cause them to lose the essen-

TEAS

Many different types of herbs are used to make teas. Some examples follow:

Flowers: Calendula chamomile, hops (strobiles), lavender, red clover, yarrow

Leaves: Basil, feverfew, ginkgo, horehound, horsetail, hyssop, motherwort, passion flower, peppermint, sage, shepherd's purse, skullcap, spearmint

Berries: Hawthorn, juniper, saw palmetto

Seeds: Fennel, milk thistle

Bark: Cinnamon, cramp bark, slippery elm

Root/Rhizome: Black cohosh, blue cohosh, burdock, dandelion, echinacea, ginger, ginseng, goldenseal, licorice, marshmallow, Oregon grape, valerian, yellow dock

Stems: Horsetail, ma huang, oat straw

tial oils. To prepare an infusion, use 1 teaspoon of dried herbs per 1 cup of hot water. (If you use fresh herbs, use 1 to 2 teaspoons or more.) Pour the hot water over the herbs in a pan or teapot, cover with a lid, and allow to steep. You can make your own herbal tea bags, too. Tie up a teaspoon of herbs in a small muslin bag (sold in most natural food stores) or piece of cheesecloth, and drop it in a cup of hot water. Let the tea steep for 15 minutes. To make larger quantities of hot infusions, use 5 tablespoons of herbs per gallon of water.

Roots, barks, and seeds, on the other hand, are best made into decoctions because these hard, woody materials need a bit of boiling to get the constituents out of the fiber. Fresh roots should be sliced thin. To prepare a medicinal use 1 teaspoon of dried herbs per cup of water, cover, and gently boil for 15 to 30 minutes. Use glass, ceramic, or earthenware pots to make your decoction: Aluminum tends to taint herbal teas and impart a bitter taste to them. Strain the decoction. A tea will remain fresh for several days when stored in the refrigerator.

To preserve teas, make a concentrated brew three times as strong as an ordinary remedy. Then add one part of drinking alcohol (*not* rubbing alcohol) to three parts of the infusion. When ready to use, dilute with three parts water.

How much of an infusion or decoction can you ingest at one time? In general, drink ½ to 1 cup three times a day. A good rule of thumb is that if you notice no benefits in three days, change the treatment or see your doctor or herbalist. Rely on professional care immediately in cases of irregular heartbeat, difficulty breathing, allergic reactions, or severe injuries.

❀ ❀ ❀

Stomach Remedy

Here's a remedy that can quiet stomach discomfort, from indigestion to a spastic colon.

1 Tbsp chamomile flowers	1 tsp fennel seeds
	2 Tbsp mint leaves

Steep 1 tsp of the mixture in 1 cup of hot water for 15 minutes; strain and drink.

❀ ❀ ❀

Coffee Substitute Decoction

If you're trying to reduce your coffee intake, this hot beverage is the perfect means to kick the caffeine habit. And if you take cream with your coffee, you can even add milk or a milk substitute such as soy or rice milk.

3 oz dandelion root	(optional)
1 oz roasted chicory root	2 oz organic orange peel
1 oz cinnamon bark	½ oz carob powder
1 oz licorice root, shredded*	1 heaping Tbsp nutmeg

Combine the herbs. Gently simmer 1 tsp of herb mix per cup of water. Lower heat, cover, and simmer for ten minutes. Turn off the heat and steep ten minutes more. Strain and drink. For a rich, sweet breakfast or dessert drink, simmer in rice milk instead of water.

*Do not use licorice if you have high blood pressure.

TINCTURES

Another popular way of making herbal medicines is to produce a tincture. Used for herbs that require a solvent stronger than water to release their chemical constituents, a tincture is an herb extracted in alcohol, glycerine, or vinegar. Tinctures can be added to hot or cold water to make an instant tea or mixed with water for external use in compresses and foot baths. The advantage of tinctures is that they have a long shelf life, and they're available for use in a pinch. You can even add tinctures to oils or salves to create instant healing ointments.

With common kitchen utensils and very little effort, you can easily prepare suitable tinctures. First, clean and pick over fresh herbs, removing any insects or damaged plant material. Remove leaves and flowers from stems, and break roots or bark into smaller pieces. Of course, you can use dried herbs, too. Cut or chop the plant parts you want to process or chop in a blender or food processor. Cover with drinking alcohol. The spirits most commonly used are 80 to 100 proof vodka or Everclear. Some herbs, such as ginger and cayenne, require the higher alcohol content to extract their constituents. With other herbs, such as dandelion and nettles, you do not need to use as much alcohol.

Puree the plant material and transfer it to a glass jar. Make sure the alcohol covers the plants. Plant materials exposed to air can mold or rot, so add more alcohol if needed. This is especially important if you use fresh herbs. Store the jar at room temperature out of sunlight, and shake the jar every-day. After three to six weeks, strain the liquid with a kitchen strainer, cheesecloth, thin piece of muslin, or a paper coffee filter. Even when you've managed to strain out every last bit of plant mate-rial, sometimes more parti-cles mysteriously show up after the tincture has been stored. There is no harm in using a tincture that con-tains a bit of solid debris. Tinctures will keep for many years without refrigeration.

Because the usual dosage of a tincture is 15 to 30 drops, you receive enough herb to benefit from its medicinal properties with very little alcohol. If you're allergic to alcohol—or simply don't wish to use it—try making vinegar- and glycerine-based tinctures. They dissolve plant constituents almost as effectively as spirits. (Glycerine is available at most pharmacies.)

❧ ❧ ❧

Dandelion Root Tincture

Place dried, chopped dandelion roots in a food proces-sor with enough 90 proof vodka to process. Once blended, store in a glass jar, shake daily, and strain in two weeks. Take $1/2$ to 1 tsp three times a day before meals for chronic constipation, poor digestion due to low levels of stomach acid, or sick headaches with nausea, or as a spring tonic.

VINEGARS

Vinegar, which contains the solvent acetic acid, is an alternative to alcohol in tinctures—especially for herbs that are high in alkaloids, which require acids to dissolve. You can use herbal vinegars medicinally or dilute them with additional vinegar to make great-tasting salad dressings and marinades. Use any vinegar with herbs, but to keep your vinegars natural, you may wish to use apple cider vinegar. Apple cider vinegar is made by naturally fermenting apple juice, while white distilled vinegar is an industrial byproduct. Rice vinegar, red wine vinegar, and balsamic vinegar are also good choices,

HERBS FOR VINEGARS		
Basil	Fennel	Raspberry
Cayenne pepper	Garlic	Rosemary
Chives	Horseradish	Tarragon
Dill	Marjoram	Thyme

but they are a bit more expensive, and their strong flavors sometimes require additional herbs.

You can apply a vinegar tincture to the skin to bring down a fever. Dilute the tincture with an equal amount of cool water. Soak a cloth in the solution and bathe the body. As the solution evaporates, it cools the body, often lowering the body's temperature by several degrees. Vinegar is also a potent antifungal agent and makes a good athlete's foot soak when combined with antifungal herbs.

❧ ❧ ❧
Foot Soak Vinegar

Place two garlic bulbs in a blender along with two handfuls of fresh or dried calendula petals, one handful of chopped fresh comfrey root, and the chopped hulls of several black walnuts (or use ½ oz black walnut tincture). Pour vinegar over the herbs and blend well. Place mixture in a large, shallow pan, and add 20 drops of tea tree oil.

To treat athlete's foot, soak feet in the solution for at least 15 minutes. Rinse feet and dry in the sun or in the light of a sun lamp. Use the foot soak three to four times a day. Make a fresh batch of the mixture for each use.

❧ ❧ ❧
Kitchen Vinegar

Not only does this preparation taste great in salads, stir-fries, and marinades, but it contains antibacterial properties as well. Gather fresh oregano and basil leaves and place in a blender with ten peeled cloves of garlic. Pour vinegar over the herbs and blend. Bottle and allow to sit for several weeks. Strain out the herbs or leave them in the preparation. For additional flavor and a nice presentation, you may add a whole sprig of oregano or basil, a cayenne pepper, and several lemon or orange rinds. This vinegar keeps well for several months unrefrigerated.

HERBAL OILS

Oils are a versatile medium for extracting herbal constituents. You may consume herbal oils in recipes or salads, or massage sore body parts with medicinal oils. To make an herbal oil, simply pour oil over herbs and allow the mixture to sit for a week or more. Olive, almond, canola, sunflower, and sesame oils are good choices, but any vegetable oil will do. Do not use mineral oil. Strain and bottle. Refrigerate oils you plan to use in cooking.

HERBS FOR OILS		
Basil	Fennel	Mint
Cayenne pepper	Garlic	Rosemary
Coriander	Ginger	Tarragon
Dill	Marjoram	Thyme

If you're watching your fat intake, place a good quality herbal oil in a small spray bottle. Before you sauté or stir-fry, spray the pan with a light film of oil. A curried peanut oil or a hot pepper sesame oil adds great taste to a stir-fry. If you need more liquid, add several tablespoons of water.

🌺 🌺 🌺

Pan Spray

Add a tablespoon of any desired powdered culinary herb to 2 ounces of peanut oil. Curry or cayenne powder are two excellent choices if you wish to add a spicy flavor to a stir-fry. Garlic, celery seed, or cumin powders are also excellent choices. Place the oil and powder in a small jar and shake daily. In several weeks, strain (a wine press works well for oils) and pour into a small spray bottle.

🌺 🌺 🌺

Massage Oil for Sore Muscles

5 or 6 cayenne peppers
  vegetable oil, about
  1 cup
¼ tsp clove essential oil

¼ tsp eucalyptus
  essential oil
¼ tsp mint essential oil

Chop cayenne peppers and place in a jar. Cover with vegetable oil; make sure the peppers are completely covered. Store oil in a warm, dark place. Strain after one week. Add the essential oils.

Massage on sore muscles. Be careful not to get this oil in your eyes or open wounds—it will sting like the dickens. Wash your hands after using this oil.

TOPICAL PREPARATIONS

It is fairly simple and lots of fun to create your own herbal skin preparations—they make great gifts, too. Commercial salves, creams, and lotions often contain byproducts and chemicals you may not wish to use on your skin. When you make your own topical preparations, you can tailor the recipes to suit your particular needs. Use your favorite kind of oil or your favorite scent. Make the lotion warming or cooling, thick or thin. There is no wrong way to make salves, liniments, or creams.

Salves

Salves, or ointments, are fat-based preparations used to soothe abrasions, heal wounds and lacerations, protect babies' skin from diaper rash, and soften dry, rough skin and chapped lips. Salves are made by heating an herb with fat until the fat absorbs the plant's healing properties. A thicken-

HERBS FOR SORE MUSCLES		
Calendula	Ginger	Lavender
Chamomile	Juniper berries	St. John's wort

HERBS THAT SOFTEN AND HEAL SKIN

Aloe vera	Comfrey	Slippery elm
Calendula	Marshmallow	

ing and hardening agent, such as beeswax, is then added to the strained mixture to give it a thicker consistency.

Kept in a cool place, salves last about six months to a year. You can preserve a salve even longer by adding a few drops of benzoin tincture, poplar bud tincture, or glycerine. (You can find benzoin tincture and glycerine in most pharmacies and poplar bud tincture in some health food stores.) Make salves in small batches to keep them fresh. Store in tightly lidded jars.

The key ingredient of salves is herbal oil. Make your oil out of the herb of your choice, as described on page 47. Calendula oil makes a wonderful all-purpose healing salve. Use St. John's wort oil to treat swelling and bruising in traumatic injuries. Use garlic oil in a salve to treat infectious conditions.

To turn the oil into a soothing salve, simply mix it with melted beeswax and allow the mixture to become solid. A general rule is to use ¾ to 1 ounce of melted beeswax per 1 cup of herbal oil. You can purchase beeswax from health food

HERBS FOR SALVES

Comfrey	Slippery elm
Goldenseal	Yarrow
Marshmallow	

stores, beekeeping supply stores, and mail-order companies. Grated beeswax melts faster. Refrigerate the wax before grating to make the job easier. You can melt the beeswax in a double boiler or in a microwave first, or add the grated beeswax to heated herbal oil—it will melt in the warmed oil. Pour the salve into containers before the blend starts to harden.

Note: Problems with your salve? Simply reheat. If your salve is too runny, add a bit more beeswax. If the salve is too hard, use more oil. To test your salve, pour about a tablespoon of salve in a container and put it in the freezer. This "tester" will be ready in a few minutes.

❧ ❧ ❧
All-Purpose Healing Salve

1 cup comfrey root oil	2 Tbsp vitamin E oil
1 cup calendula oil	20 drops vitamin A
2 oz beeswax	emulsion

Grate the beeswax. Combine the oils and gently warm them. Add the beeswax. When the beeswax is melted, add vitamins E and A. Pour into salve containers and let stand to harden.

❧ ❧ ❧
Antifungal Salve

1 cup garlic oil	2 oz beeswax
½ cup calendula oil	40 drops tea tree essential
½ tsp black walnut tincture or ½ cup oil made from black walnut hulls	oil

Grate the beeswax. Heat the garlic and calendula oils and add the beeswax. When the beeswax is melted, add the tea tree oil and black walnut tincture. Stir well. Pour into salve containers immediately.

Liniments

A liniment is a topical preparation that contains alcohol or oil and stimulating, warming herbs such as cayenne. Sometimes isopropyl, or rubbing, alcohol is used instead of grain alcohol. Do not take products made with rubbing alcohol internally.

Historically, liniments have been the treatment of choice for aching rheumatic joints and chronic lung congestion.

HERBS/ESSENTIAL OILS FOR LINIMENTS

Cayenne	Goldenseal	Rosemary
Eucalyptus	Marjoram	Wintergreen
Ginger	Peppermint	

Liniments warm the skin and turn it red temporarily. It is always a good idea to test your tolerance to a liniment by rubbing a tiny amount on your wrist to make sure it does not burn. To enhance the heat, cover the area with a cloth after application.

❧ ❧ ❧

Liniment for Arthritis, Lung Congestion, or Sore Muscles

½ oz cayenne peppers, chopped

½ oz cloves, powdered

1 oz mint leaves

1 oz eucalyptus leaves, chopped

4 cups isopropyl alcohol

60 drops essential oil of wintergreen

20 drops essential oil of peppermint

20 drops essential oil of cloves

Mix all ingredients but essential oils. Store mixture in a dark place at room temperature for two weeks. Strain or press out fluids. Add essential oils, and stir well. Massage liniment into arthritic joints, sore muscles, or onto back and chest for congestion.

Creams

A cream differs from a salve or liniment in that its liquid portion blends together with the oil. Because creams often contain water or other liquids, they are less greasy than salves and liniments. Making a cream is like making mayonnaise or gravy. Slowly add liquid to the warm wax and oil solution until the ingredients combine smoothly.

🌸 🌸 🌸
Calendula-Lavender Cream

½ tsp hydrous lanolin*
½ oz beeswax, grated
2 oz comfrey oil
2 oz calendula oil
2 oz calendula succus (fresh juice preserved with a bit of alcohol)

¹⁄₁₆ oz borax powder
¼ tsp lavender essential oil

Mix and heat oils. Melt lanolin and beeswax in the warmed oils. In another pot, gently warm succus and dissolve borax in it. Remove both mixtures from heat. Add succus to first mixture very slowly, while constantly whisking. Stir in lavender oil. Spoon into jars and seal. Cream made from fresh plant juices tends to go bad after 6 to 12 months. Store in the refrigerator.

*Hydrous lanolin is available in pharmacies.

LOTIONS

When you mix an herbal tincture or tea such as slippery elm or comfrey with an oil, it forms a thin, soothing liquid. Add essential oils for therapeutic purposes or just to create a scented lotion.

🌸 🌸 🌸
Soothing Lotion

1 oz calendula tincture
1½ oz comfrey tincture
½ oz vitamin E oil
1 oz aloe vera gel or fresh pulp

¼ tsp vitamin C crystals essential oil, if desired

Pour ingredients into a bottle and shake vigorously.

HERBS FOR COMPRESSES

Garlic	Sage
Ginger	St. John's wort
Marjoram	Witch hazel

Compresses and Poultices

You can use compresses to treat headaches, sore muscles, itching, and swollen glands, among other conditions. To make a compress, soak a cloth in a strong herbal tea, wring it out, and place it on the skin.

Soak a cloth with strong peppermint tea to treat rashes that itch and burn. Soak a cloth in cayenne powder tea to apply to an aching arthritic joint. Or soak a cloth with St. John's wort or arnica tincture and hold against a sprained ankle. A lavender or euphrasia compress can relieve itchy eyes caused by allergies.

To make a poultice or plaster, mash herbs with enough water to form a paste. Place the herb mash directly on the affected body part and cover with a clean white cloth or gauze.

HERBS FOR POULTICES

Comfrey	Oatmeal
Marshmallow	Slippery elm bark
Mustard	

Mustard Plaster

A mustard poultice is a time-honored therapy: Your great-grandmother may have used mustard poultices and plasters to treat congestion, coughs, bronchitis, or pneumonia. A mustard plaster offers immediate relief to chest discomfort and actually helps to treat infectious conditions—a much-needed therapy in the days before antibiotics. It works mainly by increasing circulation, perspiration, and heat in the afflicted area.

The person receiving the treatment should sit or lie down comfortably. The best poultices are made from black mustard seeds ground fresh in a coffee grinder, but ordinary yellow mustard powder will do in a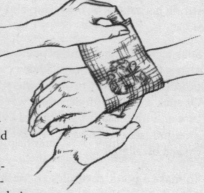
pinch. To prepare a mustard poultice, mix ½ cup mustard powder with 1 cup flour. Stir hot water into the mustard and flour mixture until it forms a paste. Spread the mixture on a piece of cotton or muslin that has been soaked in hot water. Cover with a second piece of dry material. Lay the moist side of the poultice across the person's chest or back. (She can have a second poultice on the back, or she can lie on a heating pad.)

Leave the poultice on for 15 to 30 minutes; promptly remove if the person experiences any discomfort. The procedure is likely to promote perspiration and reddening of the chest. Give the individual plenty of liquids during the procedure and encourage her to take a warm or cool shower afterward, then rest or gently stretch for a half hour.

❀ ❀ ❀

Comfrey Poultice

Use a poultice made of fresh comfrey root or leaves to help heal cuts, abrasions, and other injuries to the skin. Place comfrey in a blender with enough calendula tincture to make the blades function. Blend into a wet mass. Place the comfrey directly against the skin if there are no deep lacerations. Otherwise spread onto a muslin pad, thin layer of cheesecloth, or gauze bandage so debris won't penetrate the wound. Leave on about 30 minutes. Use the comfrey poultice several times a day for an initial injury. Poultices last several days in the refrigerator. Although comfrey helps knit many minor wounds, serious injuries should be examined by a physician.

HERBAL BATHS

Add healing herbs to baths or foot soaks; the skin absorbs the properties of many herbs. Any herb you can use to make a tea, you can use to make a bath or foot soak. Just add a pint of herbal infusion or a decoction to the water. You can also try placing herbs in a muslin bag and then suspending the bag under the hot water tap.

HERBS FOR BATHS

All-Purpose:

Lavender

Lemon balm

Rosemary

To Boost Circulation:

Ginger

Lavender

Rosemary

Yarrow

For Restful Sleep:

Chamomile

Hops

Lavender

Valerian

CAPSULES AND PILLS

We have come to rely on pharmaceutical pills to cure many of our ailments. But if you're uncomfortable with the notion of ingesting man-made chemicals, you can buy herbal capsules, tablets, and lozenges at a natural food store or make your own. Capsules and tablets also provide a convenient method of ingesting herbs that have strong, harsh flavors. People who do not enjoy drinking herbal teas or using alcohol-based tinctures may also prefer taking herbs in pill form.

Capsules

You can purchase empty gelatin capsules at health food stores, mail-order herbal houses, and some pharmacies. When making encapsulated herbs, fill one half of the capsule with the powdered herb and

pack tightly. (A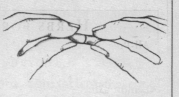
chopstick works well
to pack the pow-
dered herbs into the
capsule.) Close with
the other half of the
capsule. It takes only a couple of minutes to make
a week's supply of herbal capsules.

Pills

Blend powdered herbs with a bit of honey to bind
the mixture. Pinch off bits of the resulting sticky
substance and roll into balls. (If the balls seem too
moist, roll them in a mixture of slippery elm and
licorice powder to soak up the excess moisture.)
Dry the herbal pills in a dehydrator, an oven set to
preheat, or outdoors on a warm day covered with
a cloth. Store the dried pills in an airtight container.

🌺 🌺 🌺

Relaxation Pills

Combine equal parts of powdered skullcap, valerian,
rosemary, chamomile, and peppermint. Blend with
honey to bind. Roll off pill-sized pieces, dry, and store

A Reminder

It's best to store your herbs whole or crumbled in
large pieces. Powder them immediately before
encapsulating them. Use a mortar and pestle. For
harder roots, barks, or seeds, try powdering them in
a coffee grinder or food processor.

---

in a tightly sealed container. Use to relieve tension and calm anxiety.

Lozenges

To make herbal lozenges, combine powdered herbs with sugar and a mucilaginous binding agent such as marshmallow root, licorice root, or slippery elm bark.

❀ ❀ ❀

Throat Lozenges

3 Tbsp licorice powder*
3 Tbsp slippery elm powder
1 Tbsp myrrh powder
1 tsp cayenne powder

honey as needed
20 drops orange essential oil
2 drops essential thyme oil

Mix herbal powders. Stir in honey until a gooey mass forms. Add essential oils, and mix very well. Spread the paste on a marble slab or other nonstick surface coated with sugar or cornstarch. With a rolling pin, roll the mixture flat to about the thickness of a pancake. Sprinkle with sugar and cornstarch. With a knife, cut into small, separate squares. Or pinch off pieces and roll into ¼-inch balls. Flatten the balls into round lozenges and let dry. Allow lozenges to air-dry in a well-ventilated area for 12 hours. Suck on lozenges to help heal sore throats or coughs.

*Do not use licorice if you have high blood pressure.

SYRUPS

Made into syrups, even the most bitter herbs taste good. They're ideal for soothing sore throats and respiratory ailments. You can make herbal syrups by mixing sugar, honey, or glycerine with infusions, decoctions, tinctures, herbal juices, or medicinal liquors. (Refined sugar makes a clearer syrup with a better flavor.) To preserve syrups, refrigerate or make them with glycerine. Glycerine is often added to herbal syrups to both sweeten and preserve the mixture. Alcohol may also be added, but syrups made with glycerine are better for children.

Make syrups in small quantities. To make a simple syrup, dissolve the sweetener of your choice in a hot herb infusion. You can add herbal tinctures to increase the syrup's medicinal value: Add 1 to 2 ounces of tincture to the following formula, if you wish. Strain, if necessary, and bottle. Keep refrigerated.

❊ ❊ ❊
Herbal Syrup

¼ cup sugar or honey   1½ cups strong herb
½ cup glycerine   infusion

Combine sweetener and infusion in a pan and bring to a boil. Add glycerine. Pour into clean bottles and let cool. Keep refrigerated. Makes about 2 cups of syrup.

HERB PROFILES

❧

THIS SECTION PROFILES some of the most popular herbs in use today. You'll find these herbs in health food stores and many grocery stores. You can even grow many of the herbs yourself.

Each profile includes a description of the plant's medicinal uses along with possible side effects and precautions, and how much and what part of the plant to use to ensure safety and obtain the maximum healing potential.

The common name of the herb appears first, followed by its scientific name—the plant's genus (the first, capitalized name) and species (the second, lowercase name). It's important to identify plants by their scientific names because plants may share a common name but their uses differ significantly. Or an herb may have more than one name: Bilberry is sometimes called whortleberry. Using the genus and species names is the only way to specifically identify an herb. The herbs appear in alphabetical order by their common name.

An important note: If you use prescription medications, seek advice from a naturopathic physician or herbalist before using herbs medicinally. Blood thinning medications, in particular, may interact with herbs, other drugs, and even some foods and are the drugs most often responsible for hospitalization due to adverse side effects. Children and the elderly may require lower doses of herbs.

ALFALFA

Medicago sativa
Family: Leguminosae

❀

YOU'VE PROBABLY ENCOUNTERED alfalfa as sprouts in the produce section of your grocery store, on a sandwich, or at salad bars, but did you know the entire plant is valuable? The sprouts are a tasty addition to many dishes, and the leaves and tiny blossoms of this tall, bushy, leafy plant are used for medications.

POSSIBLE USES: Herbalists often recommend alfalfa in cases of malnutrition, debility, and prolonged illness. Alfalfa tea and capsules taken for several months build up the body. Alfalfa contains substances that bind to estrogen receptors in the body. Estrogen binds to these receptors like a key in a lock. If the estrogen level is low, and many of these "locks" are empty, the constituents of alfalfa—which resemble estrogen "keys"—bind to them instead and increase estrogenic activity. These estrogenlike keys, although similar to estrogen, are not nearly as strong. If estrogen levels in the body are too high, the alfalfa keys fill some of the locks, denying the space to estrogen, thereby reducing estrogenic activity. Because alfalfa may provide some estrogenic activity when the body's hormone levels are low and compete for estrogen binding sites when hormone levels are high, alfalfa is said to be hormone balancing.

Both alfalfa sprouts and leaf preparations may help lower blood cholesterol levels. The saponins in alfalfa seem to bind to cholesterol and prevent its absorption. Blood cholesterol levels of animals fed alfalfa saponins for several weeks have been observed to decline. Alfalfa also has been studied for its ability to reduce atherosclerosis, or plaque buildup, on the insides of artery walls. Alfalfa is high in vitamins A and C, niacin, riboflavin, folic acid, and the minerals calcium, magnesium, iron, and potassium. Alfalfa also contains bioflavonoids.

POSSIBLE SIDE EFFECTS: None reported

PRECAUTIONS AND WARNINGS: Excessive consumption of alfalfa may cause the breakdown of red blood cells. Also, a constituent in alfalfa, canavanine, may aggravate the disease lupus. Canavanine is an unusual amino acid found in the seeds and sprouts but not in the mature leaves. Thus, alfalfa tea and capsules made from leaves would not contain canavanine. Avoid alfalfa during pregnancy because of its canavanine content and hormonally active saponins. If you are pregnant, you may put a few sprouts on a sandwich now and then, but avoid daily consumption of alfalfa.

PART USED: Leaves, small stems, and young flowers

ALFALFA SPROUTS

Treat yourself to alfalfa sprouts you've grown yourself. Alfalfa seeds are inexpensive; you can purchase them in a health food store. Place 2 tablespoons in the bottom of a 1-quart canning jar. Soak the seeds in water overnight. Place a piece of fine-mesh cheesecloth over the top of the jar and secure it with the canning lid. Strain the soaking water and rinse the seeds several times with clean water. Position the jar at a 45-degree angle and leave the jar tilted downward so water can drain and air can circulate. Rinse the seeds each morning and evening, and they will sprout in two to five days, depending on the temperature and seed quality. When sprouts are 1 inch long, with tiny leaves forming, place the jar in a window for another day or two. Continue to rinse the seeds twice a day as the leaves turn green, then take the sprouts from the jar and store them in the refrigerator.

PREPARATION AND DOSAGE: Alfalfa is available in capsules, which you may take daily as a nutritional supplement. You can also find bulk alfalfa leaves, which you can infuse to make a nourishing tea.

Capsules: Take 1 or 2 capsules a day.

Tea: Infuse 1 tablespoon per cup of boiling water and steep for 15 minutes. You may drink several cups a day. Add lemon grass, mint, or other flavorful herbs to improve the taste.

ALOE VERA
Aloe barbadensis (formerly *Aloe vera*)
Family: Liliaceae

*A*LMOST EVERYONE is aware of the healing virtues of aloe vera. This well-known medicinal plant is used around the world to treat skin ailments and burns. Aloe is commercially cultivated in warm and tropical climates, namely Barbados, Haiti, Venezuela, and South Africa, and warm regions of the United States, such as Texas. But all you need is a warm area to grow your own potted aloe plant.

POSSIBLE USES: Aloe is cherished for its wound healing and pain relieving effects. Many people keep an aloe plant in their kitchens so it is readily available to treat burns from grease splatter or hot utensils. (Severe burns require treatment by a physician.) Aloe is even safe for use on children.

Aloe contains slippery, slimy constituents that have a demulcent, or soothing effect. An early study published in the *International Journal of Dermatology* in 1973 describes the effects of aloe vera gel topically on leg ulcers. Each of the three patients studied had a serious raw, open sore on the leg for 5 to 15 years. (These ulcers commonly occur in individuals with diabetes, those who have problems with blood circulation, and those who are bedridden.) After aloe was repeatedly applied to the ulcers, the ulcers healed completely in two patients; the third patient's ulcer showed significant improvement. More recent studies have also shown aloe to have similar wound healing abilities.

Scientists are investigating the use of aloe in treating cancer and certain blood diseases, particularly those associated with low white blood cell counts such as leukemia. In fact, veterinarians use extracts from the aloe plant to treat cancer and feline leukemia in their animal patients. It is thought that a molecule, known as acemannan, in the aloe gel stimulates the body to produce disease-fighting white blood cells, particularly macrophages. The word macrophage means "big eater"—macrophages engulf and digest unwanted substances, such as bacteria and viruses, in the bloodstream and tissues. Macrophages also release substances that battle tumor cells and fight infection.

POSSIBLE SIDE EFFECTS: None

PRECAUTIONS AND WARNINGS: Health food stores sometimes carry aloe vera juice for oral consumption, claiming it relieves gastrointestinal complaints such as indigestion. Such claims are

Aloe Body Rub

Treat yourself to a soothing body rub. Simply scrape the moist pulp from the inside of a succulent aloe vera leaf and mash it with a fork. Apply the preparation to your skin, and wash it off after 20 minutes. You can also slice aloe leaves lengthwise and use their inner sides as a body scrub in the shower.

questionable at best, thus it's wise to limit aloe vera to external use, particularly if you are pregnant or have one of the following conditions: gastritis, heartburn, irritable bowel syndrome, ulcerative colitis, Crohn disease, or hemorrhoids.

Aloe vera juice is sometimes recommended as a laxative. While aloe does contain a purgative agent (an agent that stimulates bowel movements), the bowels may become dependent on aloe vera juice used regularly to regulate the bowels. If you experience constipation, take a close look at your diet. If increased fiber and water intake do not improve the problem, consult your physician.

PART USED: Mucilage in leaves

PREPARATION AND DOSAGE: To treat a burn, slice a plump aloe leaf lengthwise, and apply it directly to the skin. You can also scrape out the leaf's inner pulp, mash it with a fork, and apply the moist gel to the burn. A wide variety of commercial aloe preparations, including gels, soaps, skin creams, and burn remedies, are also available.

BILBERRY
Vaccinium myrtillus
Family: Ericaceae

THOUGH YOU MAY NOT
recognize the name,
you are already familiar
with the *Vaccinium* genus of
herbs. It includes numerous
plants that bear small,
round, dark blue or dark purple
edible berries. Blueberries, huckleberries, and bilberries are three of
more than 100 species of the *Vaccinium* genus
found throughout the United States and Europe.
If you eat whortleberries and creme in England,
you're getting a healthy dose of bilberries.
Bilberries and huckleberries are popular food for
hikers and forest birds and animals. The berries
also make good dyes (with alum as a mordant)
and very tasty jellies and jams. These berries freeze
quite well, so you can harvest them in the summer
and store them for year-round consumption.

POSSIBLE USES: Both the leaves and the ripe
fruit of the bilberry and related berry species have
long been a folk remedy for treating diabetes.
Traditionally, people used the leaves to control
blood sugar. While the leaves can lower blood
sugar, they do so by impairing a normal process in
the liver. For this reason, use of the leaves is not
recommended for long-term treatment.

The berry, on the other hand, is recommended for people with diabetes. The berries do not lower blood sugar, but their constituents may help improve the strength and integrity of blood vessels and reduce damage to these vessels associated with diabetes and other diseases such as atherosclerosis (calcium and fat deposits in arteries). The berries contain flavonoids, compounds found in the pigment of many plants. The blue-purple pigments typical of this family are due to the flavonoid anthocyanin.

With their potent antioxidant action, anthocyanins protect body tissues, particularly blood vessels, from oxidizing agents circulating in the blood. In the same way pipes rust as a result of an attack by chemicals, so various chemicals in our environment—pollutants, smoke, and chemicals in food—can bind to and oxidize blood vessels. Two common complications of diabetes, diabetic eye disease (retinopathy) and kidney disease (nephropathy), often begin when the tiny capillaries of these organs are injured by excessive sugar deposits. Antioxidants allow these harmful oxidizing agents to bind to them instead of to body cells.

Bilberries also help keep platelets from clumping together, which thins the blood, prevents clotting, and improves circulation. Bilberry preparations seem particularly useful in treating eye conditions, so in addition to their use with diabetic retinopathy, they are also used to treat cataracts, night blindness, and degeneration of the macula, the spot in the back of the eye that enables sharp focusing.

POSSIBLE SIDE EFFECTS: None reported

PRECAUTIONS AND WARNINGS: People with insulin-dependent diabetes should not use bilberry leaves. The leaves do not have the beneficial flavonoid-related effects of the berries, and they contain properties that irritate the liver. Use of the berries is appropriate because they do not interfere with diabetes medications, and they can help prevent some complications of diabetes.

PART USED: Ripe berries

PREPARATION AND DOSAGE: You can simply add bilberries, blueberries, and huckleberries to your diet. Teas and tinctures are usually made from the leaf; these products should not be used long-term or by persons with diabetes. The berry is also available as bilberry extract. For treatment of eye conditions, it's best to purchase a *Vaccinium* product.

🌹 🌹 🌹

Bilberry Jam

4 cups clean, picked-over, ripe berries	Juice of 1 lemon
2 cups honey	1 package pectin

Mix ingredients in a pan. Simmer one hour, removing any foam that rises to the surface. Stir in pectin, mix thoroughly, and pour into jam containers. Store opened jam in the refrigerator.

BLACK COHOSH

Cimicifuga racemosa
Family: Ranunculaceae

❦

POSSIBLE USES: If you ache—whether from menstrual cramps, an injury, or a condition such as rheumatism—black cohosh may be the herb you need. Black cohosh acts as an antispasmodic to muscles, nerves, and blood vessels and as a muscle anti-inflammatory. It contains the anti-inflammatory salicylic acid (the ingredient in aspirin), among other constituents, and has been used for a variety of muscular, pelvic, and rheumatic pains. It seems particularly effective for uterine cramps and muscle pain caused by nervous tension and pains accompanied by stiffness, soreness, and tight sensations of contraction. Native Americans used it for female and muscular conditions, and early American physicians used black cohosh for female reproductive problems, including menstrual cramps and bleeding irregularities, as well as uterine and ovarian pain.

Black cohosh is used as an emmenagogue, an agent that promotes menstrual or uterine bleeding. Herbalists consider it a sedative emmenagogue, meaning it promotes blood flow when uterine tension, cramps, and congestion hinder flow. Black cohosh relaxes the uterus, especially when tension is caused by anxiety. Black cohosh is believed to act on the uterus by improving muscle tone, so it is useful for preventing miscarriage and premature labor. The herb is also recommended for women who have had difficult labors; it is administered in small doses in the last trimester of pregnancy to prepare the uterus for delivery. It decreases labor pain by promoting more efficient contractions. When contractions during labor are weak, or for severe afterpains following labor, black cohosh is used.

The herb is also thought to have an estrogenic effect because its constituents bind to estrogen receptors in the body. The binding of a plant constituent to an estrogen receptor can increase estrogen activity in the affected tissues. This hormonal activity may improve uterine problems, such as poor uterine tone, menstrual cramps, and post-menopausal vaginal dryness. One recent study evaluated the effects of black cohosh and a placebo in 110 menopausal women. The women were given 8 milligrams of black cohosh or the placebo every day for eight weeks, and then blood levels of hormones were checked. The results showed that black cohosh has an estrogenic effect, and it could particularly benefit postmenopausal women.

Black cohosh is also a mild stomach tonic credited with alterative action. (An alterative is an agent capable of improving the absorption of nutrients and the elimination of wastes by the digestive tract.) Its sweet and bitter flavors stimulate digestion. Black cohosh has been shown to dilate peripheral blood vessels and sometimes improve elevated blood pressure. Early physicians also used black cohosh for serious infectious diseases, including whooping cough, scarlet fever, and smallpox. In China, the Chinese species, *Cimicifuga foetida,* is used for measles.

POSSIBLE SIDE EFFECTS: Some people who react to salicylate-based medicines, such as aspirin, may experience ringing in the ears or asthmatic wheezing when they take black cohosh. The herb may promote blood flow to the head, resulting in a sensation of fullness and, occasionally, headache. Dizziness, nausea, and slow pulse rate are reported rarely. Avoid black cohosh if you are pregnant unless it is specifically indicated and prescribed by a naturopathic physician.

PRECAUTIONS AND WARNINGS: Do not take black cohosh for head pain that is full or pounding because black cohosh mildly increases blood flow to the head.

PART USED: Root

PREPARATION AND DOSAGE: Black cohosh is available in tincture or capsule form.

Capsules: Take 2 to 4 per day.

Tincture: Take ¼ to ½ teaspoon two to four times daily.

BLUE COHOSH
ALSO CALLED BLUE GINSENG, SQUAW ROOT, PAPOOSE ROOT
Caulophyllum thalictroides
Family: Berberidaceae

*E*ARLY AMERICANS LEARNED from the native peoples to use blue cohosh as a women's herb. So impressed were the pioneer physicians by this Native American medicine, they listed blue cohosh as an official medicine in the U.S. Pharmacopoeia.

POSSIBLE USES: Blue cohosh is used primarily for uterine weakness and as a childbirth aid. It is considered a uterine stimulant in most circumstances, improving uterine muscle tone; yet it also has an antispasmodic effect on cramps. Because of its dual actions, herbalists describe blue cohosh as a uterine tonic. The alkaloid methylcytisine found in blue cohosh is thought to be antispasmodic, while the triterpenoid saponin hederagenin is thought to provide the increased uterine tone.

Blue cohosh is also classified as an emmenagogue, meaning it stimulates menstrual flow. It dilates blood vessels in the uterus and promotes circulation in the pelvis, making it helpful for women who experience scanty, spotty menstrual flow; irregular periods; and difficult, painful periods. Blue cohosh seems to work best for women who experience more painful menstrual cramps the first day of their period. You may use blue cohosh to relieve menstrual cramps and to treat a weak, worn-out, or sluggish-acting uterine muscle—indicated by no cramps or weak cramps but prolonged bleeding; weak pelvic, abdominal, and thigh muscles; and an aching, dragging sensation during the menstrual period. Blue cohosh also may be useful in cases of breast tenderness and abdominal pain caused by fluid retention.

Blue cohosh helps correct uterine prolapse (sagging of the uterus in the pelvic cavity). This condition may stem from multiple childbirths or tissue laxity due to overweight or obesity. Blue cohosh also may help the uterus shrink back to its appropriate size after childbirth.

The herb has long been used by herbalists to prepare the uterus for childbirth. It is often combined with other botanicals (historically, black cohosh, motherwort, and partridge berry). The formula is taken in the last trimester of pregnancy to promote smooth, efficient labor and delivery, and rapid involution of the uterus (returning of the uterus to its normal size). While some sources state that blue cohosh is contraindicated during pregnancy, many herbalists and women have used blue cohosh safely and effectively during late pregnancy. This herb should not be used during early pregnancy, and it should be used during late pregnancy only under the supervision of a physician or skilled herbalist.

Blue cohosh is a diuretic, an agent that promotes urination, and a weak diaphoretic, an agent that raises body temperature and promotes sweating, which may help break a fever.

POSSIBLE SIDE EFFECTS: Large, repeated doses (a dropper full of tincture every hour) may irritate the throat. Soreness subsides quickly once you stop taking the medication. Nausea, headache, and elevated blood pressure have also been reported with these large, frequent doses. The plant's tempting blue berries should not be eaten raw; they won't kill you, but they could make you sick. Cooked berries are not thought to be toxic.

PRECAUTIONS AND WARNINGS: Because of its alkaloids, blue cohosh should not be used for longer than four to six months. The alkaloid methylcytisine may elevate blood pressure in susceptible individuals when used regularly for longer than this. Blue cohosh should not be used during pregnancy, except in the last month or two, and then only under the advice of a physician or skilled herbalist.

PART USED: Root

PREPARATION AND DOSAGE:

Tea: Boil 1 ounce of dried root per 2 cups of water. Drink ¼ to ½ cup two to four times a day.

Tincture: Take 10 to 30 drops of tincture at a time, one to six times a day.

BURDOCK

Arctium lappa, Arctium minus
Family: Compositae

*H*AVE YOU EVER RETURNED from a romp with your dog and found burrs on your clothing and in your pup's fur? Then you've literally come in contact with burdock. *Arctium* bears its seeds in the form of small spherical burrs, hence the name burdock. Close examination of a burdock burr reveals a small hook on the end of its tiny spikes. These hooks catch on the fur of passing animals or on the clothes of passing people, thus dispersing the plant's seeds. Burdock was the inspiration for Velcro fasteners!

POSSIBLE USES: Burdock is a perennial whose roots, and sometimes its seeds, are used widely in herbal medicine to support liver function and as a cleansing botanical. Like dandelion and yellow dock, burdock roots are bitter and thus capable of stimulating digestive secretions and aiding digestion. These roots are referred to as alterative agents—capable of enhancing digestion and the absorption of nutrients and supporting the elimination of wastes. Any botanical capable of these important actions can attain far-reaching improvements in a variety of complaints.

Burdock may also be useful to treat a variety of skin conditions, including acne and dryness of the skin, especially when these complaints are due to poor diet, constipation, or liver burden. The liver plays an important role in removing impurities from the blood, producing bile to digest fats, metabolizing hormones, and storing excess carbohydrates. Everything absorbed from the digestive tract goes directly to the liver to be filtered, so when you eat foods that contain pesticides, preservatives, artificial coloring and the like, you give your liver extra work to do. A high fat diet also forces your liver to work harder because it must break down the fats with the bile it produces. Add to this all of the potential toxins we are exposed to in daily life that the liver must also remove from the bloodstream (car exhaust, nicotine, prescription drugs, alcohol, cleaning products, industrial toxins, etc.), and you can see how the liver can become overworked or burdened.

When the amount of toxic substances in a person's bloodstream exceeds the liver's capacity to remove them from circulation, the offending substances get stored in the body. The accumulated toxins are stored in body fats primarily, but they can produce numerous symptoms, including headaches, acne, itching, chronic gas and indigestion, nausea, arthritis, and other complaints. For this reason, many herbalists and naturopathic physicians recommend internal use of alterative herbs for these chronic conditions.

Burdock is also useful in cases of hormone imbalance that have not been attributed to uterine fibroids, cancer, or other diseases. Many conditions such as PMS, fibroids, and endometriosis are associated with excess estrogen levels. Because of its alterative action, and because of the small amounts of plant steroids it contains, burdock can help improve the liver's ability to metabolize hormones such as estrogen and thereby improve symptoms associated with hormonal imbalance.

Burdock contains a starchlike substance called inulin. Burdock has been recommended to people with diabetes because studies show inulin is easier for their system to metabolize than other starches.

POSSIBLE SIDE EFFECTS: Due to its ability to promote digestive acid and secretions, burdock can cause heartburn and a sour stomach in rare instances.

PRECAUTIONS AND WARNINGS: If you have ulcers, an irritable bowel, or excessive stomach acid, burdock may worsen your condition. Burdock and all the alteratives may still be appropriate under certain circumstances, but you should consult an experienced herbalist before using them. Avoid burdock, or any substance that increases stomach acid, during a bout of diarrhea, ulcer flare-up, or case of heartburn.

PART USED: Roots primarily, sometimes seeds

PREPARATION AND DOSAGE: You can eat burdock, tincture it, or dry it for use in teas or capsules. Roots are available in the produce section of many grocery stores in the fall as gobo root, the Japanese name for burdock. You should see positive effects of its use within three weeks; use it for two to three months. It makes a good coffee substitute. To improve digestion, take the tea or tincture 15 to 30 minutes before a meal.

Tea: Drink 2 to 4 cups per day.

Tincture: Take ½ to 1 teaspoon three or four times a day.

❀ ❀ ❀

Gobo Root Stir-Fry

Burdock or gobo root, sliced thin

1 large, yellow onion, chopped

2 large carrots, sliced thin

1 red bell pepper, sliced thin

15–20 shiitake or common mushrooms, sliced

1 Tbsp ginger root, grated

1 cup peanuts

Sesame oil (about 2 Tbsp)

⅓ cup soy or tamari sauce

¼ cup honey

Sauté the burdock, carrots, and onions in sesame oil on low heat for 5 minutes. Add peanuts and sauté 5 to 10 minutes more. Add the red pepper and mushrooms, soy sauce, and honey; reduce heat as low as possible. Cover for 10 minutes, stirring occasionally. Serve over brown rice.

CALENDULA, POT MARIGOLD

Calendula officinalis
Family: Compositae

POSSIBLE USES:
Calendula has a long history of use as a wound healing and skin soothing botanical. This lovely marigold-like flower (although called pot marigold, it is not a true marigold) is considered a vulnerary agent, a substance that promotes healing. Calendula also has anti-inflammatory and weak antimicrobial activity. It is most often used topically for lacerations, abrasions, and skin infections, and less commonly internally to heal inflamed and infected mucous membranes.

Numerous topical preparations exist for external use. Calendula salve, for example, is a useful and versatile product to keep in the first aid kit or home medicine chest. In addition to its use to treat minor cuts and abrasions, the salve is great for chapped lips and diaper rash. You can use calendula teas as a mouthwash for gum and tooth infections, a gargle for sore throats and tonsillitis, a vaginal douche for infections and irritation, and a sitz bath for genital inflammation or hemorrhoids. Or drink the tea to help treat bladder infections or stomach ulcers.

POSSIBLE SIDE EFFECTS: None commonly reported; calendula is considered safe and nontoxic.

PRECAUTIONS AND WARNINGS: Do not apply any fat-based ointments, including calendula salve, to wounds that are oozing or weeping; use watery preparations only such as calendula tea, and allow the area to air-dry completely between applications. On recently stitched wounds, wait until stitches have been removed and scabs have formed before applying calendula ointments or other preparations to severe lacerations or injuries. An exception would be a very brief and light application of calendula succus or tea applied without any rubbing or friction.

PART USED: Flowers and, occasionally, leaves

PREPARATION AND DOSAGE: Most health food stores carry calendula soaps, oils, lotions, salves, and creams. Herb stores also supply bulk dried flowers, tincture, and calendula succus, which is made by extracting the fresh juice from the leaves and young flowers and preserving it with a bit of alcohol. Calendula succus is popular among naturopathic physicians who use it during minor surgical procedures (to help heal the incision) and topically on skin wounds and infections.

CALENDULA IN THE KITCHEN

Calendula is extremely easy to grow and will flower abundantly for many months, even in cold climes, so a gardener will have a steady supply of the useful flowers. In most regions, calendula reseeds itself, producing crops year after year. Pull the petals from the flower heads or cut with scissors and add to salads, pastas, rice, and other whole grains. Add the petals after dishes are already cooked—simply stir in at the last minute before serving. The petals are palatable and offer vibrant, interesting color to many recipes. You can also add the petals to salad dressings and sauces, or float them atop soups.

Tincture: For internal use, take 1 teaspoon, three or more times daily. You can also use the tincture to make a salve.

Tea: Infuse 1 heaping tablespoon of dried flowers per cup of hot water. Drink 2 to 4 cups each day.

To use calendula tea topically, soak a clean cloth in the tea and apply it to the skin.

CAYENNE PEPPER
Capsicum annum
Family: Solanaceae

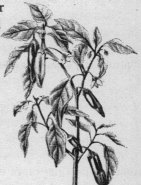

*A*RE YOU A HOT SALSA or chili fan? Then you'll want to learn more about the virtues of hot peppers. These ripe fruits of the *Capsicum* genus are widely used as a popular spice, but hot peppers are also dried and powdered or tinctured for medicinal purposes.

POSSIBLE USES: Cayenne stimulates digestion and muscle movement in the intestines, which helps restore deficient digestive secretions and aids absorption of food nutrients. (Stomach acid tends to decline with age, and some cases of poor digestion are related to this lack of acid.) Cayenne also stimulates circulation and blood flow to the peripheral areas of the body. Because of its ability to stimulate digestion and circulation, cayenne is often added to a wide variety of herbal remedies: It improves the absorption and circulation of the other herbs throughout the body.

Have you ever gone after the chips and salsa with gusto and then felt flushed and drippy in the nose? Cayenne warms the body and stimulates the release of mucus from the respiratory passages. Anyone who has eaten much cayenne knows hot peppers can clear the sinuses and cause sweating. Cayenne can actually raise the body temperature a bit as it stimulates circulation and blood flow to the skin. An herb, such as cayenne or ginger, that promotes fever and sweating has a diaphoretic action. This action can help "break a fever" and relieve colds and congestion.

Fever is a natural and necessary phenomena generated by the body to fight bacteria and viruses. It is a misconception that fever is harmful or undesired; only very high or prolonged fevers are dangerous. Fevers speed up metabolic processes to increase production of disease-fighting white blood cells.

Cayenne has become a popular home treatment for mild high blood pressure and high blood cholesterol levels. Cayenne preparations prevent platelets from clumping together and accumulating in the blood, allowing the blood to flow more easily. Since it is thought to help improve circulation, it's often used by those who have slow metabolisms due to low thyroid function or those who are always cold or have cold hands and feet.

You can use cayenne peppers topically as a pain-relieving muscle rub and joint liniment. The source of their heat is capsaicin, the fiery phenolic resin found in most hot peppers. Capsaicin causes nerve endings to release a chemical known as substance P. Substance P transmits pain signals from the body back to the brain. When capsaicin causes substance P to flood out of the cells, we experience a sensation of warmth or even extreme heat. When the nerve endings have lost all of their substance P, no pain signals can be transmitted to the brain until the nerve endings accumulate more substance P. For this reason, topical cayenne pepper products are popular for the treatment of arthritis and bursitis and for temporary relief of pain from psoriasis, herpes zoster, and neuralgia (nerve pain). These cayenne preparations are most appropriate for longstanding chronic conditions, not acute inflammations.

Cayenne is often found in diet and weight-loss formulas. But can eating hot peppers really help you lose weight? Probably not, but cayenne may promote calorie burning, supporting your diet and exercise efforts. Because it aids in digestion and absorption of nutrients, cayenne can reduce appetite that is due to malabsorption, a common condition in overweight people.

PRECAUTIONS AND WARNINGS: If you've ever accidentally rubbed your eyes after cutting hot peppers, you know you should respect this herb. Cayenne pills may cause a burning sensation in the throat, stomach, or rectum of some sensitive individuals. Some people may tolerate liquid cayenne preparations or combination products better than tablets or capsules. Others may find cayenne pepper in the diet easier to digest than cayenne medications. Use small, cautious doses only. Avoid getting cayenne into the eyes or open wounds. Do not use topical applications of cayenne products too frequently, as there is some concern that nerve damage could occur with daily repetitive use. Cayenne placed directly on the skin can cause burns and even blisters, so dilute a cayenne preparation in oil before placing it on the skin, or mix it with flour and water until it forms a paste, which you can spread on muslin to prepare a poultice. You can also mix cayenne with orris root powder and dust it very lightly on heavily oiled skin, working it in with massage.

Do not use in cases of high fever of 104 degrees Fahrenheit or above. Cayenne preparations are not recommended for use by individuals who have rapid heart rates or who become overheated or perspire easily.

POSSIBLE SIDE EFFECTS: Cayenne peppers are a member of the Solanaceae, or Nightshade, family, which includes tomatoes, potatoes, eggplant, and tobacco. Some individuals have an intolerance to this entire family, experiencing symptoms, often joint pain, after eating even a small amount of these foods.

PREPARATION AND DOSAGE: To clear a head cold and relieve sinus pain and congestion, try drinking a cup of tea made with lemon and ginger or horseradish to which you've added a dash or two of cayenne pepper.

Cayenne Sore Throat Gargle

Use this gargle to relieve sore throats, hoarseness, and respiratory congestion.

⅛ to ½ tsp cayenne (depending on individual tolerance), powdered

2 Tbsp salt

10 drops mint essential oil

10 drops orange oil

2 drops thyme essential oil

2 drops myrrh essential oil

Bring 2 cups of water to a boil. Reduce heat, add salt and cayenne, and simmer 15 minutes. Stir vigorously, and add oils.

Use 1 cupful to gargle with. Rinse out mouth with plain water, and repeat with the second cup of gargle solution.

TAKE THE TASK TEST

When cooking or making medicines with cayenne peppers, you must take into account the widely varying intensities of different peppers—from very mild to extremely fiery. There is even considerable variance in heat of peppers from the same bush throughout the season or due to the health and size of the pepper. Always taste peppers first and use them accordingly.

CHAMOMILE, GERMAN
Matricaria recutita
(formerly *Matricaria chamomilla*)
Family: Compositae

*P*ETER RABBIT'S MOTHER gave him chamomile tea when he was feeling poorly, and maybe your mother brewed you a cup of this soothing tea to help ease your tummy troubles, too. Chamomile, indeed, is an excellent choice for stomach aches. Several different plants are called chamomile but not all belong to the *Matricaria* genus. English or Roman chamomile *(Chamaemelum nobile,* formerly *Anthemis nobilis)*, for example, is a different species, yet it shares many of German chamomile's chemical constituents and, therefore, many of its actions. (Now you can see why botanists always use Latin names to discuss plants.) Though they may have very different Latin names, if the plants have the same taste, color, and aroma as *Matricaria recutita*, they likely have a similar action.

POSSIBLE USES: The genus *Matricaria* is derived from the Latin matrix, meaning womb, most likely because chamomile is widely used to treat gynecologic complaints. Chamomile has been found to contain fairly strong antispasmodic and anti-inflammatory constituents and is particularly effective in treating stomach and intestinal cramps.

Chamomile reduces cramping and spastic pain in the bowels and also relieves excessive gas and bloating in the intestines. It is often used to relieve irritable bowel syndrome, nausea, and gastroen-teritis (what we usually call stomach "flu"). Chamomile is also an excellent calming agent, well suited for irritable babies and restless children; it can also help a child fall asleep. Moreover, most children tolerate its taste. Chamomile is calming to adults as well, so don't hesitate to sip it throughout the day. It is an ideal choice for those with ulcers or other stomach problems aggravated by anxiety.

Muscle pain that results from stress and worry is another indication for chamomile. Twitching and tics in muscles may respond to chamomile tea or other chamomile medications.

Chamomile is valued as an antimicrobial agent. A German study found that the herb inactivates bac-terial toxins. Small quantities of chamomile's oil inhibit staphylococcal and streptococcal strains of bacteria. You can drink chamomile tea combined with other antimicrobials such as thyme, echi-nacea, and goldenseal for internal infections. You can use chamomile topically, too, to treat infec-tions and inflammations. Although the plant contains not a hint of blue, chamomile contains a potent volatile oil that is a brilliant blue when isolated. This oil, called chamazulene after its dark azure color, has strong anti-inflammatory actions. Apply a preparation made from its volatile oil to skin infections, or apply cloths soaked in strong chamomile tea to eczema patches and other inflamed skin surfaces. Small children with eczema, bug bites, or diaper rash may take a bath of warm chamomile and oatmeal tea.

POSSIBLE SIDE EFFECTS: Most people tolerate chamomile well. You don't need to reserve chamomile for medicinal purposes. It can be drunk as a beverage—even by the young and old. Many herbalists advise pregnant women to avoid using any herbs they don't really need, but chamomile shouldn't cause a problem if used occasionally.

PART USED: Tops gathered in the early stages of flowering

PREPARATION AND DOSAGE:

Tea: Steep 1 tablespoon of chamomile flowers per cup of water for 15 minutes. Drink a half cup up to five times a day for digestive problems. For nervous conditions, combine chamomile with equal parts of passion flower, skullcap, oats, or hops.

Tincture: Take 30 to 60 drops, three times per day.

❧ ❧ ❧
Stomach and Bowel Tea

This all-purpose stomach tea is useful for nausea, spastic colon, irritable bowel, ulcers, and colitis. Omit the licorice if you have high blood pressure.

German chamomile flowers	Fennel seeds
Licorice root, shredded	Peppermint

Combine equal parts of dry herbs, and steep 1 tablespoon of the mixture in a cup of hot water for 15 minutes. Strain and drink 2 or more cups a day as needed for gastrointestinal problems. This tea is quick acting, even for long-standing problems. You should notice effects within several hours for acute ailments and within several days for chronic conditions such as spastic colon or ulcers.

❧ ❧ ❧
Teething Baby Tea

You may give chamomile to teething infants to calm them and reduce gum inflammation. If a child will not drink chamomile tea from a bottle or take it from a spoon, soak a cloth in ½ cup of strong chamomile tea to which you've added 2 drops of clove oil. Place the cloth-tea mixture in the freezer for 20 minutes, then give to the baby to chomp on.

CHASTE TREE

Vitex agnus castus
Family: Verbenaceae

POSSIBLE USES: *Vitex* was used by men in the Middle Ages to diminish their sex drive, and its common names, chaste tree and monk's pepper, stem from its use by monks to maintain celibacy. Researchers are unsure about chaste tree's effects on women's libidos; although it does seem to reduce sex drive in women, the effects are less pronounced than in men.

In modern times, chaste tree is used primarily as a women's herb for menstrual complaints. The flavonoids in chaste tree exert an effect similar to the hormone progesterone, although the plant contains no hormonal compounds. Many menstrual complaints are known to result in a relative lack of progesterone. When progesterone levels are low relative to estrogen, infertility, heavy bleeding, lack of periods, too-frequent periods, irregular periods, and PMS can result. Because it helps increase progesterone levels, chaste tree alleviates these complaints. It can normalize and regulate menstrual cycles, reduce premenstrual fluid retention, and treat some cases of acne that flare up during menstruation. Chaste tree can also be used for menopausal bleeding irregularities, such as frequent or heavy bleeding; it is often combined with dong quai or wild yam.

Chaste tree is slow-acting and can take months to produce effects. When treating infertility, chaste tree is used for one to two years; it is discontinued if pregnancy occurs. The effects are gentle and gradual; it gradually increases progesterone levels, allowing normal ovulation and pregnancy.

POSSIBLE SIDE EFFECTS: The strong bitterness of chaste tree may be nauseating to some. Rarely, chaste tree may cause heavier menstrual flow.

PRECAUTIONS AND WARNINGS: There are no known dangers, but you should not use this or any herb unless you need to. Because of its complex hormonal actions, chaste tree is not recommended for use during pregnancy.

PART USED: Berries

PREPARATION AND DOSAGE: Chaste tree berries are typically tinctured or powdered and used in capsule form. The flavor is rather unpleasant, so chaste tree is not a popular tea.

Tincture: Take ¼ to ¾ teaspoon one to three times daily, and reduce dosage when effect is noted. Although effects can be more rapid, it may take three months before you see improvements.

Capsules: Take 2 to 3 capsules a day.

CINNAMON

Cinnamomum saigonicum (Saigon Cinnamon)
Cinnamomum zeylanicum (Ceylon Cinnamon)
Family: Lauraceae

POSSIBLE USES: You probably have some cinnamon powder or sticks in your kitchen cupboard. Cinnamon is a warming, stimulating, pleasant-tasting herb with many uses. Cinnamon is widely used as a flavoring agent for candy, toothpaste, mouthwashes, and bath and body products. In herbal teas, cinnamon improves the flavor of less palatable herbs. And, of course, it is a staple for baking and cooking.

Perhaps you use cinnamon more in the winter. Spiced cider, prepared by steeping cinnamon sticks and other herbs in apple cider, is a traditional winter beverage. Cinnamon has an affinity for the uterus and digestive organs because it improves circulation and energy flow in the abdomen. In Chinese medical philosophy, pain, cramps, and congestion are considered blocked energy. Cinnamon is thought to circulate qi, or vital energy, when it is stuck in the abdomen and move it to the rest of the body and to warm the body.

Cinnamon has a germicidal effect. Almost all highly aromatic herbs display some ability to kill germs and microbes. Cinnamon in mouthwashes and gargles can help kill germs and treat infections.

You may use small amounts of cinnamon tea to relieve gas in the stomach. Larger amounts of cinnamon will stimulate and warm the stomach, promoting acidity and a laxative effect. Use of cinnamon as a laxative may prevent flatulence and intestinal cramping that can accompany use of some other laxatives.

POSSIBLE SIDE EFFECTS: Some people may experience a warming sensation or sweating, and some may experience headaches, nausea, or diarrhea after ingesting two or more cupfuls of a strong cinnamon tea or spiced cider. Cinnamon used regularly may, in rare cases, elevate blood pressure in some people. If you are prone to high blood pressure or if you already have high blood pressure, consult with an herbalist before using cinnamon tea or tincture on a daily basis. Cinnamon in your apple pie or sweet roll is unlikely to cause problems with elevated blood pressure; however, cinnamon is an herb that many people with irritable bowel conditions and allergies may react to. If you have a fever or diarrhea caused by irritation or stimulation in the intestines such as with stomach "flu," food poisoning, irritable bowel, or colitis, cinnamon may worsen the condition. (Most sudden-onset, acute episodes of diarrhea are due to inflammation, irritation, or infection, and a strong dose of cinnamon could further stimulate the bowels.) If you have a severe irritable bowel, a bowl of cinnamon-flavored cereal could have a laxative effect.

PRECAUTIONS AND WARNINGS: Avoid if you have a high fever, are red and sweating, or have uncontrolled high blood pressure or irritable bowels. If you have multiple allergies or sensitivities, use cinnamon cautiously. If you're pregnant, you may use cinnamon in baking, but avoid more than a cup of cinnamon tea at a time.

PART USED: Bark

PREPARATION AND DOSAGE: Dried bark is ground into fine powder or cut into small chunks for decoctions and drunk as a tea.

Tea: Boil 1 teaspoon of dried bark in a cup of hot water, and drink 1 or 2 cups when needed. If you tend to have heavy periods, drink several cups of cinnamon tea a day before or during your period.

Tincture: Take 10 to 60 drops at a time, usually combined with other herbs. Use the higher doses for a menstrual period that is much heavier than usual.

Essential oil: The volatile oil from cinnamon is distilled and used as a flavoring and aromatic agent. Use a single drop of cinnamon essential oil diluted in a sip of water as a mouth rinse to freshen your breath and for mouth and gum infections. Use 8 to 10 drops of cinnamon essential oil in a 2-ounce tincture bottle for flavor or medicinal effects. Keep essential oils out of your eyes.

❦ ❦ ❦
Spiced Cider

1 gallon apple cider	5 whole cloves
5 cinnamon sticks	1 tsp nutmeg
3 star anise	1 or 2 oranges
5 whole allspice kernels	

Blend cinnamon, star anise, allspice, cloves, and nutmeg into apple cider in a large pot. Use a zester or grater to remove the rind of the oranges and add to the cider mix. You can also cut the rind (taking care to remove any pith), and grind it in a blender with a bit of the cider; then add it to the pot. Add the juice of the oranges to the cider. Heat to just below simmer for several hours. Ladle into mugs and serve with a cinnamon stick.

COMFREY
Symphytum officinale
Family: Boraginaceae

❧

POSSIBLE USES: Comfrey is from the Latin *conferta,* meaning "to grow together"; *Symphytum* means the same in Greek. Comfrey is so named because of its use to knit bones, mend lacerations, and heal wounds.

Comfrey has been found to cause cells to divide at an increased rate, thereby healing bones and wounds more quickly. Comfrey may be used topically on cuts, bruises, abrasions, and burns. The internal use of comfrey has sparked much debate among herbalists. Most health regulatory agencies in the Western world have banned the internal use of comfrey. Cases of poisoning and even one death have been documented from internal use of comfrey. Comfrey contains pyrrolizidine alkaloids, which are known to harm the livers of animals fed diets consisting largely of comfrey leaves. Most herbalists recommend other herbs for internal use.

The problems generally arise from long-term use of the herb—four months or more. A medical professional may prescribe comfrey for short-term use, while carefully supervising the patient. But you should never use comfrey internally on your own. Technically, *Symphytum officinale* is not the culprit; *Symphytum uplandicum,* or Russian comfrey, is the unsafe herb. However, the two are used interchangeably in the U.S. marketplace, and there's no way to tell which herb you've gotten.

POSSIBLE SIDE EFFECTS: Liver damage has been reported with repeated internal use.

PRECAUTIONS AND WARNINGS: Do not use comfrey internally. Comfrey is safe to use topically even on infants, the elderly, or pregnant women.

PART USED: Root

PREPARATION AND DOSAGE: Use comfrey root for topical teas and tinctures. You can also use the raw root topically. While teas are easy to prepare, comfrey is a bit tricky to tincture; it tends to mold. Mucilaginous herbs are best extracted with a low alcohol percentage (around 45 percent). Apply cold grated comfrey root or a cloth soaked in cool comfrey tea to sunburns or other minor burns. Apply comfrey poultices to wounds.

COMFREY OIL

Clean fresh comfrey roots with a scrub brush under running water. Place the roots in a blender or food processor with olive oil to cover, and grind as fine as possible. Transfer to a large glass jar and allow to soak for several weeks before straining. Use as a compress or poultice.

CRAMP BARK

Viburnum opulus
Family: Caprifoliaceae

❦

POSSIBLE USES: You may be familiar with this low-growing shrub with thick shiny leaves and, on some species, dark shiny berries. Dense, compact, and attractive, it is often used as ornamental shrubbery, but this beautiful shrub is also valuable medicinally. As its name implies, cramp bark is useful to ease uterine cramps. But as a muscle relaxant, it also affects other organs, including the intestines and the skeletal muscles.

Cramp bark is considered the most potent uterine antispasmodic of the various *Viburnum* species because it contains more of the antispasmodic constituent scopoletin. It also contains more anti-spasmodic volatile oils than other species. Cramp bark usually works rapidly for simple menstrual cramps. If the herb fails to relieve symptoms, the discomfort is probably not due to uterine muscle spasm but to inflammation or irritation of uterus or ovaries, endometrial infection, or cysts. Cramp bark's close relative, black haw, is also useful for uterine cramps, congestion, and irritation and radiating pains in the uterus and ovaries. Black haw contains an anti-inflammatory constituent as well and may be better indicated for those types of complaints.

Cramp bark has been used to halt contractions during premature labor. It has also been used in the last trimester of pregnancy to build up uterine muscles and ensure an easy labor. A formula known as Mother's Cordial was used in early American medicine to facilitate childbirth because of its muscle-strengthening effect on the uterus. Mother's Cordial may help pregnant women who experience uterine or pelvic cramps and weakness due to multiple childbirths. Consult with an experienced herbalist or naturopathic physician before taking any botanicals during pregnancy.

The antispasmodic constituents in cramp bark also may lower blood pressure by relaxing vessel walls. When taken in large dosages (30 drops or more every two or three hours), cramp bark may reduce leg cramps, muscle spasms, or pain from a stiff neck.

POSSIBLE SIDE EFFECTS: Nausea, vomiting, and diarrhea have been reported with large doses of 60 drops or more taken hourly. Even this large dose, however, is often tolerated with no side effects or problems. People sensitive to aspirin may also be sensitive to cramp bark.

PRECAUTIONS AND WARNINGS: Cramp bark is harmless in regular doses. Do not use if you have a sensitivity to aspirin.

PART USED: Root, dug in summer or fall

PREPARATION AND DOSAGE: Bark is peeled from the root and dried for decoctions or made into an alcohol or glycerine tincture.

Tea: Drink 3 or more cups a day for stomach cramps.

Tincture: A typical dosage is 30 to 60 drops an hour for acute muscle spasm. (A naturopathic physician might prescribe 60 drops of cramp bark tincture every half hour for obstetrical emergencies such as a threatened miscarriage.) For dysmenorrhea (painful menstruation), cramp bark seems to work best when taken frequently. Start with ½ dropper (⅛ teaspoon) very half hour until an effect is noted, then every one to three hours. Reduce the dosage as symptoms abate.

If your menstrual cycles are regular, you can use a cramp bark preparation three to four times a day starting the day before the usual onset of cramps. Don't take cramp bark during the entire cycle for menstrual cramps, however; use it as you need it.

❀ ❀ ❀
Mother's Cordial

Combine equal parts of tinctures of cramp bark, blue cohosh, black cohosh, and false unicorn root. Take ½ to 1 teaspoon two to three times a day during the last trimester.

DANDELION
Taraxacum officinale
Family: Compositae

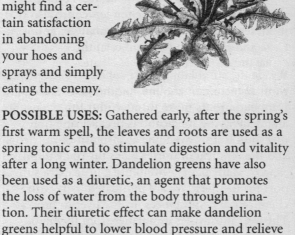

DID YOU KNOW an extremely useful medicine and food already grows in your yard? In fact, if you've spent countless hours battling your dandelions, you might find a certain satisfaction in abandoning your hoes and sprays and simply eating the enemy.

POSSIBLE USES: Gathered early, after the spring's first warm spell, the leaves and roots are used as a spring tonic and to stimulate digestion and vitality after a long winter. Dandelion greens have also been used as a diuretic, an agent that promotes the loss of water from the body through urination. Their diuretic effect can make dandelion greens helpful to lower blood pressure and relieve premenstrual fluid retention.

Dandelion roots contain inulin and levulin, starch-like substances that may balance blood sugar, as well as a bitter substance (taraxacin) that stimulates digestion. The very presence of a bitter taste in the mouth promotes the flow of bile from the liver and gallbladder, and hydrochloric acid from the stomach. Bitters have been used for centuries in many countries before meals as a digestive stimulant. Do you avoid bitter-tasting foods? Many people do, but this may not reflect a balanced appetite. According to Asian philosophies, the diet should contain foods that are sweet, salty, sour, and bitter. The few bitter tastes Westerners embrace are coffee, wine, and beer, which may have something to do with the higher incidence of digestive diseases in Western cultures compared with Asian cultures. Dandelion leaves are also rich in minerals and vitamins, particularly vitamins A, C, K, and riboflavin (B_2) and calcium.

Beside the stimulating bitter substances, dandelion roots also contain choline, another liver stimulant. Dandelion roots make wonderful colon cleansing and detoxifying medications because any time digestion is improved, the absorption of nutrients and the removal of wastes from the body improves as well. Many people could use a little extra support for the liver: We are inundated daily with chemicals and substances for the liver to process. The liver must filter impurities from the bloodstream—all the car exhaust, paints, cleaners, solvents, preservatives, pesticide residues, drugs, alcohol, and other toxins we encounter can begin to tax the liver. Add a diet high in fat, which the liver must emulsify with bile, and a person could experience physical symptoms of this burden on the liver. Rough, dry skin and acne, constipation, gas and bloating, frequent headaches, and PMS are all potential symptoms of liver burden.

Dandelions are also recommended for wart removal. The roots, stems, and leaves of the dandelion exude a white sticky resin when injured. Applied directly to warts daily or, preferably, several times a day, this resin slowly dissolves them.

POSSIBLE SIDE EFFECTS: Side effects are uncommon, but intestinal irritation and loose bowels can occur with use of the root.

PRECAUTIONS AND WARNINGS: In certain situations, stimulating digestive secretions is not advisable, so dandelion should be used in small amounts only or not at all. So avoid dandelion use if you have diarrhea, hyperacidity (too much stomach acid), ulcers, irritable bowel, or ulcerative colitis, particularly during a flare-up of these conditions. Persons prone to gallstone flare-ups should avoid dandelion since it promotes the gallbladder to contract and secrete bile and could possibly worsen an inflammation. Dandelion is probably safe for individuals with "silent" gallstones, that is, those that show up at X-ray or ultrasound examination but do not cause any symptoms.

PART USED: Entire plant—roots, leaves, and flowers

PREPARATION AND DOSAGE: You can eat dandelions prepared fresh from your yard or you can dry and tincture them. If you want to use your own dandelions, don't use any chemical sprays on your lawn (a good idea in any case), and be wary where you gather dandelions.

Tea: Drink several cups of dandelion tea made from the root or the leaf daily. To make diuretic teas, herbalists prefer using dandelion leaves rather than roots.

Tincture: Take 1 to 2 teaspoons daily, all at once or in smaller doses throughout the day.

❧ ❧ ❧

Dandelion Juice Spring Tonic

Make a cleansing, nourishing juice from the dandelions you weed out of your lawn. The sweetness of the apples and carrots improves the bitter taste of the dandelion. Consume this preparation in small quantities as a spring tonic.

3 cups dandelion roots	6 organic apples,
10 organic carrots, sliced	quartered

In a home juicer, juice the dandelion roots, carrots, and apples separately. Combine the juices in a blender and chill 30 minutes to allow flavors to blend. Blend with any of the following: 1 tsp vitamin C crystals, 1 tsp spirulina powder, ¼ tsp liquid multiminerals.

To treat colds and congestion, add garlic, cayenne, or horseradish, and sip the tonic throughout the day.

❀ ❀ ❀
Sautéed Greens

Gather young dandelion leaves in the spring, and add them to soups or stir-fry, or steam them. Or sauté them with mushrooms, onions, and shredded kale and cabbage in a bit of sesame oil. The greens cook quickly, even on low heat, so take care not to overcook. (Overcooked greens are mushy.) Remove from heat, and add a dash of toasted sesame oil and balsamic vinegar, and garnish with sesame seeds. Serve as a side dish or with a sauce over rice.

❀ ❀ ❀
Dandelion Wine

The day before you make the wine, place wine yeast in a large jar with a bit of warm water and the juice from a lemon slice. Stuff a paper towel in the top of the jar and set it aside.

On the day you make the wine, purée 1 pound of dandelion flowers with 2 cups of water. Place the purée in a large bucket; add 2 pounds of sugar and 3½ quarts of boiling water. Mix until the sugar dissolves. When the mixture cools to 100° F, add the yeast, cover, and store in a warm place for ten days, stirring each day.

After ten days, strain, and place the liquid in a large bottle such as an empty apple cider jug. Place an air-lock on the jug. Bind a plastic bag to the airlock to trap gases given off during the fermentation process. When no more gas inflates the bag, siphon the wine. Bottle, cork, and store it for at least six months.

DONG QUAI, ANGELICA
(ALSO KNOWN AS DANG GUI, TANG KUEI, AND TANG KWEI)
Angelica sinensis
Family: Umbelliferae

❀

*L*EGEND HAS IT that angelica received its name after an angel revealed herself to a medieval European monk and taught him the medicinal virtues of angelica. *Angelica sinensis,* commonly called dong quai, is native to China and has been used there as a medicine for thousands of years. This botanical is now commonly used in North America as well. Dong quai has a faint anise-like flavor; the seed oil is sometimes extracted and used as a flavoring. (The leaves of the European species, *archangelica,* flavor the liqueur Benedictine.) Dong quai preparations are readily available in health food stores and many regular grocery stores.

POSSIBLE USES: Dong quai is used primarily to treat menstrual complaints, such as painful flow and scanty or excessive menstruation. Studies have shown that dong quai is useful in treating other gynecologic complaints as well, including infertility, premenstrual syndrome (PMS), menstrual cramping and irregular cycles, chronic miscarriage, and menopausal complaints. Dong quai's strong effect on the female reproductive organs is similar to that of steroids or hormones: It is believed to enhance the function of uterine and ovarian cells.

Though dong quai does not actually contain steroids or hormone molecules, one of its consituents is coumarin. Coumarin is most widely known for its use in preventing blood clotting, but constituents related to it may have numerous actions. For example, these compounds bind to the same areas on body membranes that estrogen compounds do—areas called estrogen receptors. During menopause, the levels of estrogen produced by the ovaries decline and result in symptoms such as hot flashes. Since the coumarin compounds in dong quai act like estrogen, they can help reduce symptoms that occur as a result of declining estrogen levels. Many women report that use of dong quai eases menopausal symptoms, including hot flashes.

Dong quai also contains ferulic acid, a pain reliever and muscle relaxer. Indeed, the herb is often used to treat painful menstrual cramps or other cases of uterine spasms. Oddly enough, several studies have shown that dong quai acts as a muscle relaxant overall, but before it relaxes the uterus it stimulates the uterus briefly. The uterus is a muscle, and when dong quai stimulates it, its tone improves and it becomes tight and contracts more readily. All muscles function better when they are well toned, and the uterus is no exception. A well-toned, strong, healthy uterus is less prone to cramps and muscle spasm. In addition to relaxing the uterus, ferulic acid may also relax the heart muscles, lower blood pressure, and calm cardiac arrhythmias (a variation in the normal rhythm of the heartbeat).

Studies also cite dong quai's effectiveness in treating allergies and respiratory complaints. Several chemical agents in dong quai may have an antihistamine and antiserotonin effect. Histamine, serotonin, and other substances are released from blood cells in response to something that irritates the body—pollen, dust, chemical fumes, animal dander, to name a few—and causes the symptoms we associate with allergies. An antihistamine curbs these symptoms, thus dong quai's reported antiallergy effects.

POSSIBLE SIDE EFFECTS: Dong quai is considered quite safe, though it may make some people's skin more sensitive to sunlight. You should avoid prolonged sun exposure while using dong quai preparations.

PRECAUTIONS AND WARNINGS: Because dong quai dilates the blood vessels and improves circulation in the uterus, regular use can sometimes make menstrual flow heavier—in China, dong quai is called a "blood mover." Many herbalists recommend that use of dong quai be stopped during the actual menstrual period in women prone to heavy flow or if heavy bleeding is a concern. These women can use a separate formula such as cramp bark or cinnamon bark during their menstrual period and dong quai during the rest of the cycle. Also, because dong quai is warming and stimulating, the Chinese warn against its use in people prone to "heat signs": hot face or hands, thirst, dry throat and lungs, fast pulse, and insomnia. Do not use dong quai if you take blood thinning or high blood pressure medication. Also avoid in pregnancy.

PART USED: Root (You can use the leaves, stem, and seeds as a confection and a flavoring agent.)

PREPARATION AND DOSAGE: Dong quai can be dried and made into a tincture or powdered and encapsulated.

For menstrual cramps: Take a dropper full of dong quai tincture every one to three hours, starting the minute you feel the cramps coming on. If your periods are regular, you might start the day before your period is due or the day before the expected onset of the cramps.

For relief of menopausal symptoms: Take 1 or 2 dong quai capsules at a time or 1 or 2 droppers (½ to 1 teaspoon) of tincture at a time three times a day. If after a week, you notice no or limited improvement in symptoms, increase the dose to four, five, or even six times a day. Most people need a higher dosage of three to six times per day. Once they achieve relief, many women are able to cut the dosage back down after a month or so without diminishing the effect. You should begin noticing effects in one or two weeks.

❧ ❧ ❧
Candied Angelica Stems

A close American relative of dong quai is garden angelica, *Angelica archangelica*. You can prepare a candied treat from its stems.

Slice the hollow stems into thin strips. Immerse them in boiling water for three to five minutes. Remove and quickly plunge them into ice cold water for several minutes. Spread the slices on a paper towel to dry for several hours. Dip each slice in a bowl containing whipped egg white and lemon juice, and transfer to a sheet of wax paper. Sprinkle each slice with sugar and allow the egg white to absorb it. Flip the slices over and repeat. Continue sprinkling sugar every few hours until the egg white is saturated with sugar and begins to crystallize. Transfer to a clean sheet of wax paper and store in a small, covered container.

These treats will keep indefinitely. Eat them as is or use them to decorate frosted cakes and cookies.

ECHINACEA, PURPLE CONEFLOWER

Echinacea purpurea
Family: Compositae
Related Species: *Echinacea angustifolia*

❧❀

POSSIBLE USES: If you've ever walked into a health food store or herb store and asked for something to treat your cold, you probably received an echinacea product. The roots and sometimes leaves of this beautiful sunflower family member make an important medicine used widely to treat colds, flu, bronchitis, and all types of infections. Native to prairies and temperate woodlands throughout the United States, this showy perennial was used by the Native Americans and adopted by the early settlers as a medicine. Members of the medical profession in early America relied heavily on echinacea, but it fell from favor with the advent of pharmaceutical medicine and antibiotics. Many physicians are returning to echinacea today. Many forms of echinacea are available to choose from; Germany has registered more than 40 different echinacea products. Echinacea is entering the world of big business with vast acres of cropland devoted to cultivating and processing this prominent herbal medicine.

Echinacea is used primarily to boost the immune system and help the body fight off disease. In addition to increasing many chemical substances that direct immune response, echinacea increases both the number and the activity of white blood cells; raises the level of interferon, a substance secreted by blood cells that enhances immune function; and stimulates blood cells to engulf invading microbes. What all this means is that under the influence of echinacea, white blood cells become more active and more likely to seek out and destroy offending substances. Echinacea also increases the production of substances the body produces naturally to fight cancers and speeds removal of pollutants from the lungs.

Besides its use as an immune stimulant, echinacea is recommended for individuals with recurring boils and as an antidote for snake bites.

POSSIBLE SIDE EFFECTS: Echinacea is considered quite safe, even at high and frequent doses, and may be used by children and the elderly without worry in almost all cases. The question has been raised whether echinacea could be harmful for people with autoimmune or overactive immune diseases, such as lupus or rheumatoid arthritis. Currently, there is no evidence that echinacea is either helpful or harmful.

Frequent use of echinacea may mask the symptoms of a more serious underlying disease. If you have any persistent condition, consult a physician.

PRECAUTIONS AND WARNINGS: Due to their medicinal value, many tons of the roots are sold annually; thus, echinacea species are disappearing from the wild. As with many botanicals, it might be best to grow your own echinacea or purchase it from a reputable herb source that cultivates its own herbs and not from people who harvest echinacea from its native habitat.

PART USED: Root and leaves

PREPARATION AND DOSAGE: Echinacea is not terribly tasty in a tea, unless you add other, more palatable, herbs. For this reason, echinacea is most often taken as tincture or as pills. However, liquid preparations—teas and tinctures—appear to be more effective than the powdered herb in capsules. If you take the capsules, first break them open and put them in a little warm water and drink the water. Most herbalists recommend large and frequent doses at the onset of a cold, flu, sinus infection, bladder infection, or other illness.

For acute infection: Take a dropper full of tincture every one to three hours, or 1 to 2 capsules every three to four hours for the first day or two, reducing the dosage thereafter.

For a chronic infectious problem: Take echinacea three times a day for several months on and then several weeks off.

FENNEL
Foeniculum vulgare
Family: Umbelliferae

❧

POSSIBLE USES: This familiar culinary herb is considered a digestive aid and gas reliever. It is recommended for numerous complaints related to excessive gas in the stomach and intestines, including indigestion, cramps, and bloating, as well as for colic in infants. An agent capable of diminishing gas in the intestines is called a carminative. Other Umbell family members such as dill and caraway are also considered carminatives.

As an antispasmodic, fennel acts on the smooth muscle of the respiratory passages as well as the stomach and intestines, so fennel preparations are used to relieve bronchial spasms. Because it relaxes bronchial passages, allowing them to open wider, it is sometimes included in asthma, bronchitis, and cough formulas.

Fennel is also known to have an estrogenic effect and has long been used to promote milk production in nursing mothers.

POSSIBLE SIDE EFFECTS: Although a few rare individuals may experience allergic reactions to fennel, it is generally considered quite safe and nontoxic. Pregnant women should not consume large amounts of fennel tea or take any other fennel preparations, as it could cause their milk to come in too early.

PRECAUTIONS AND WARNINGS: None cited

PART USED: Leaves, seeds

PREPARATION AND DOSAGE: Fennel seeds are most commonly used as medicine and a cooking spice. For the best effect and flavor, crush the seeds a bit before using them.

❀ ❀ ❀

Quinoa Salad with Orange Fennel Dressing

1 cup quinoa

3 cups water

1 carrot, grated

2 cups peas, fresh or frozen

½ cup purple onion, chopped

2 cups arugula, shredded

½ cup nuts (walnuts, almonds, or pine nuts)

1 orange

2 Tbsp maple syrup

2 Tbsp sesame oil

1 Tbsp balsamic vinegar

½ tsp cumin

2 heaping Tbsp fresh fennel greens (or 1 Tbsp ground fennel seeds)

Boil quinoa in water until soft. Drain and place in a salad bowl with carrots, peas, onion, and arugula. Chill. Place 1 to 2 Tbsp orange zest in a blender. Add the orange, taking care to remove any pith. Add maple syrup, sesame oil, balsamic vinegar, cumin, and fennel. Purée. Toss in salad with nuts, and serve.

FEVERFEW

Tanacetum parthenium
Formerly: *Chrysanthemum parthenium,*
Pyrethrum parthenium
Family: Compositae

*F*EVERFEW IS INDIGENOUS to Europe and the Balkan peninsula and is said to have grown around the Greek Parthenon, thus the species name *parthenium*. Feverfew has made its way to both North and South America, where it is now naturalized.

POSSIBLE USES: Feverfew is used to relieve headaches, particularly vascular headaches such as migraines. Doctors aren't sure what causes migraines, but they know these severe headaches involve blood vessel changes. One theory is migraines occur when the blood vessels in the head expand and press on the nerves, causing pain. Another theory is these headaches occur as the blood vessels react to outside stimuli by affecting blood flow to various parts of the brain. Feverfew relaxes tension in the blood vessels in the brain and inhibits the secretion of substances that cause pain and inflammation (such as histamine and serotonin). Studies confirm feverfew's effectiveness as a migraine remedy.

Although some herbalists believe feverfew is most effective when used long-term to prevent chronic migraines, some people find it helpful when taken at the onset of a headache. Besides vascular headaches, feverfew may also benefit those who experience premenstrual headaches, which are often due to fluid retention and hormonal effects.

Feverfew is also reported to reduce fever and inflammation in joints and tissues. Some physicians recommend it to relieve menstrual cramps and to facilitate delivery of the placenta following childbirth.

Feverfew contains the substance parthenolide, which has been credited with inhibiting the release of serotonin, histamine, and other inflammatory substances that make blood vessels spasm and become inflamed. Reportedly, the amount of parthenolide varies from plant to plant, so it is wise to know how much of this active ingredient a feverfew product contains before you buy it. One study of commercially available feverfew products found that most of them contained no parthenolide at all: They were dried herbs, and because parthenolide is volatile, it had all evaporated. Look for a product that contains 0.2 percent parthenolide.

POSSIBLE SIDE EFFECTS: Feverfew can cause stomach upset. Chewing the raw leaves day after day can irritate the mouth; the irritation subsides once you stop chewing the leaves. Tinctures and capsules do not irritate the mouth.

Since feverfew relaxes blood vessels, it can increase blood flow during menstruation and possibly even induce abortion if taken in early pregnancy. Keep feverfew out of reach of children. Study is still needed to determine the herb's safety long-term. Extreme overdose may induce a coma or even be potentially fatal due to respiratory failure.

PRECAUTIONS AND WARNINGS: Feverfew is sometimes called tansy, but do not confuse fever-few (*Tanacetum parthenium*) with the herb tansy (*Tanacetum vulgare*) or with various *Senecio* species commonly known as the ragworts, which are also sometimes referred to as tansy. You can see the value of botanical versus common names here. Avoid feverfew in pregnancy because it may induce abortion of the fetus.

PART USED: Leaves, primarily

PREPARATION AND DOSAGE: Feverfew is dried for tinctures, capsules, and infusions or simply eaten fresh. Since feverfew is a lovely garden plant and easy to grow, many herbalists recommend that people who experience chronic headaches plant it in their yards where it is readily available.

The dosage of feverfew depends on the type and quality of the product used. Consuming two to three of the bitter tasting raw leaves each day constitutes a medicinal dosage. Limit consumption to a maximum of four or five leaves a day. If mouth irritation occurs, eat only one leaf at a time; place it in a salad or sandwich to reduce irritation.

Tea: Prepare an infusion using about 1 tablespoon of dried leaves per cup of hot water; steep for ten minutes.

Capsules: Take 1 to 3 per day.

Tincture: Take 10 to 20 drops daily to prevent headache or every half hour at the onset of a migraine. For arthritis and joint inflammation, take a larger dose of 30 to 40 drops two to three times daily.

GARLIC

Allium sativum
Family: Liliaceae
Related Genus: *Allium cepa* (Onion)

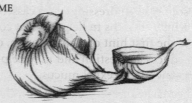

GARLIC'S RESUME would read something like this: cholesterol lowerer, blood pressure reducer, blood sugar balancer, cancer combatant, fungus fighter, bronchitis soother, cold curer, wart remover, and immune system toner. And don't overlook garlic's previous employment as a vampire deterrent or its potential career as an organic pesticide.

With a resume like this, it's no wonder garlic has gained such popularity with advocates of herbal medicine. It is one of the most extensively researched and widely used of all plants. Its actions are diverse and affect nearly every body tissue and system. Garlic preparations abound in health food stores. Lots of people include garlic in their daily diet for health reasons, while many others eat it because they love its pungent flavor. Many thousands of acres are devoted to the cultivation of garlic in the United States alone. If you drive through Gilroy, California, in the summer with your windows down, you can believe this town's claim to be the garlic capital of the world.

POSSIBLE USES: As an antimicrobial, garlic seems to have a broad action. It displays antibiotic, antifungal, and antiviral properties and is reportedly effective against many flu viruses and herpes simplex type I strains (the virus responsible for cold sores). You may add garlic liberally to soups, salad dressings, and casseroles during the winter months to help prevent colds, or eat garlic at the first hint of a cold, cough, or flu. Garlic reduces congestion and may help people with bronchitis to expel mucus.

Garlic is used to treat many types of infections: Use capsules internally for recurrent vaginal yeast infections, or use a garlic infusion topically as a soak for athlete's foot or add to an oil to treat middle ear infections.

This popular herb may improve immunity by stimulating some of the body's natural immune cells. Studies suggest that garlic may help prevent and treat breast, bladder, skin, and stomach cancers. A recent study of women in Minnesota suggests that women who eat garlic may lower their risk of colon cancer. Garlic appears particularly effective in inhibiting compounds formed by nitrates, preservatives used to cure meat that are thought to turn into cancer-causing compounds within the intestines.

Garlic lowers blood pressure by relaxing vein and artery walls. This action helps keep platelets from clumping together and improves blood flow, thereby reducing the risk of stroke. Garlic also decreases the level of LDL (low-density lipoprotein, or "bad" cholesterol).

Garlic contains a large number of rather unique sulfur-containing compounds, which are credited with many of garlic's medicinal actions. Did you ever wonder why garlic bulbs on your kitchen counter don't smell strongly until you cut them? That's because an enzyme promotes conversion of alliin to the odorous allicin. Allicin and other sulfur compounds are potent antimicrobials and thought to have blood purifying and, possibly, anticancer effects.

The constituents in garlic also increase insulin levels in the body. The result is lower blood sugar. Thus garlic makes an excellent addition to the diet of people with diabetes. It will not take the place of insulin, antidiabetes drugs, or a prudent diet, but garlic may help lower insulin doses.

POSSIBLE SIDE EFFECTS: Some individuals are sensitive to garlic and cannot use it in large amounts without feeling nauseous and hot. Others don't digest sulfur compounds well, and gas and bloating result. Garlic used topically, such as in eardrops for ear infections, can irritate skin and membranes in sensitive people.

PRECAUTIONS AND WARNINGS: If you know that too much garlic upsets your stomach, don't eat it or ingest it as a medicine. If you're not sure, use garlic cautiously at first to determine how well you tolerate it.

PART USED: Bulb

PREPARATION AND DOSAGE: Garlic is available fresh, dried, powdered, and tinctured. In health food stores, garlic appears primarily in capsule form or combined in tablets with other herbs. Since garlic's antibiotic properties depend on odorous allicin, deodorized garlic preparations are not effective for this use. The label of such products may identify them as having a particular "allicin content," but they remain ineffective as antibiotics. Deodorized products are quite effective for lowering blood pressure and cholesterol, however. Of course, the tastiest way to get your dose of garlic is to add it liberally to your diet. Brushing your teeth or nibbling on fresh parsley after eating garlic can help keep you socially acceptable.

Capsules: Take 800 mg a day.

Tincture: Take 1 or 2 droppers (¼ to ½ teaspoon) in a glass of water, two to four times daily. For painful ear infections, place 1 or 2 drops of warm garlic oil in the ear canal several times a day at the onset of ear pain.

Infusion for topical use: Crush a garlic bulb and steep in 4 to 5 cups of hot water. Soak feet in the preparation for 15 to 20 minutes up to three times a day to treat athlete's foot.

🌸 🌸 🌸
Roasted Garlic

Peel two bulbs of garlic and combine in a small roasting dish with sliced red bell pepper, a grated carrot, and a small amount of peanut oil. Place underneath the broiler for two or three minutes, stir the pepper and carrot, and return for two or three minutes more. The bulbs should become slightly browned. Eat small amounts frequently at the onset of a cold or a flu for a natural antibiotic effect.

🌸 🌸 🌸
Garlic Soup for Colds and Flu

8 cups water

2–3 Tbsp miso (a salty fermented soybean product available in health food stores)

3 carrots, sliced

1 white onion, chopped

2 Tbsp ginger root, grated

1 bunch kale, washed and shredded

1 bulb garlic, peeled and crushed

Place carrots, onion, ginger root, and miso in the water and simmer until onions are translucent and carrots begin to get soft. Add garlic and kale, reduce heat to lowest possible setting, and warm for another hour. Drink the soup during the day, eating little else.

GINGER
Zingiber officinale
Family: Zingiberaceae

❦

*T*HIS BOTANICAL and popular spice is native to southeast Asia but is readily available in the United States. Fresh ginger root is a staple in Asian cooking. Dried and powdered, it's used in medicine. Ginger is high in volatile oils, also known as essential oils. Volatile oils are the aromatic part of the plants that we so cherish. They are called volatile because as unstable molecules, they are given off freely into the atmosphere.

POSSIBLE USES: Ginger root powder may be useful in improving pain, stiffness, lack of mobility, and swelling. Larger dosages in the area of 3 or 4 grams of ginger powder daily appear most effective. But powder may not be the only effective form of ginger root: One study demonstrated benefits from the ingestion of lightly cooked ginger.

Ginger has also had a long history of use as an antinausea herb recommended for morning sickness, motion sickness, and nausea accompanying gastroenteritis (more commonly called stomach "flu"). As a stomach calming aid, ginger also reduces gas, bloating, and indigestion, and aids in the absorption and the body's use of other nutrients and medicines. It is also a valuable deterrent to intestinal worms, particularly roundworms. Ginger may even improve some cases of constant severe dizziness and vertigo. It may be both a therapy and a preventive treatment for some migraine headaches. Ginger also prevents platelets from clumping together in the bloodstream. This serves to thin the blood and reduce the risk of atherosclerosis and blood clots.

A warming herb, ginger can promote perspiration when ingested in large amounts. It stimulates circulation, particularly in the abdominal and pelvic regions, and can occasionally promote menstrual flow. If you are often cold, you can use warm ginger to help raise your body temperature.

When used topically, ginger stimulates circulation in the skin, and the volatile oils absorb into underlying tissues. You may want to try ginger root poultices on the chest for lung congestion or on the abdomen for gas and nausea. Powdered ginger and essential oils are the strongest form of ginger for topical use.

POSSIBLE SIDE EFFECTS: Since ginger can warm and raise body temperature slightly, it should be avoided when this is undesired, such as in someone with menopausal hot flashes.

PRECAUTIONS AND WARNINGS: Avoid ginger preparations for fevers that are over 104 degrees

Fahrenheit. Although ginger is recommended for morning sickness, those with a history of miscarriage should avoid it. Since ginger stimulates blood flow and thins the blood, promoting uterine bleeding is a concern. Some people actually become nauseous if they consume a large quantity of ginger; for others, ginger relieves nausea. It is best to use ginger cautiously at first.

PART USED: Root

PREPARATION AND DOSAGE:

Capsules: For nausea, take 1 to 2 capsules every two to six hours. To alleviate arthritis pain, try higher dosages of 15 to 25 capsules per day.

Tea: Drink 1 or 2 cups of ginger tea to promote a warming effect. To promote actual perspiration, you'll need more.

🌺 🌺 🌺
Warming Tea

10–12 thin slices of fresh ginger root
4 cups of water
Juice of 1 orange

Juice of ½ lemon
½ cup honey or maple syrup (optional)

Place ginger root and water in a pan, and boil gently for 10 minutes. Strain. Add orange juice, lemon juice, and honey. Consume as a warming tea. Several large cups consumed in a row or drunk in a hot bath can elevate the body temperature and promote perspiration. This sweating therapy may help break a fever or reduce congestion.

❧ ❧ ❧
Candied Ginger Throat Lozenges

Fresh ginger root,
  sliced ¼-inch thick
½ cup honey
Thyme essential oil
Orange essential oil

Mint essential oil
Eucalyptus essential oil
Licorice powder
Slippery elm powder

Simmer ginger root in water until just soft (about
½ hour). Dry briefly on paper towels. To ½ cup of
honey, add 10 drops of each of the oils, and stir. Dip
the ginger slices into the honey mixture and place on
wax paper. Mix licorice and slippery elm powders in
equal proportions. Dust the ginger slices with the powder
mixture over several days until the powder no longer
absorbs. Store the lozenges in an airtight container or
wrap them individually. Suck on them for throat pain
and coughs.

❧ ❧ ❧
Ginger Poultice for Congestion

Grate 1 whole ginger root into a bowl. Stir in ¼ tsp of
cayenne oil or powder and 2 drops of thyme essential
oil. Place a coat of plain oil or ointment on the skin to
be treated. For swollen tonsils and enlarged lymph nodes
in the neck, oil the neck, throat, and underside of the
chin. For bronchitis and lung congestion, oil the upper
chest and back. Spread the grated ginger root mixture on
the skin and cover with a sheet of plastic wrap. Cover
this with a heating pad or hot, moist towel. Leave in
place for 15 to 30 minutes. The skin will become red and
warm, but you should not feel any pain. Remove the
poultice promptly if you feel any discomfort. For infants
and adults with sensitive skin, omit the cayenne and
thyme oil.

GINKGO
Ginkgo biloba
Family: Ginkgoaceae

❧

*T*HE LOVELY GINGKO tree is the oldest living species of tree. Once it may have covered the globe, but it nearly became extinct after the Ice Age and survived only in parts of Asia. Ginkgo was a favorite plant of Chinese monks, who cultivated the tree for food and medicine.

The ginkgo tree now has established itself as a useful urban landscape plant, gracing city streets and parks. Because ginkgo is resistant to drought, disease, and pollution, it can live as long as a thousand years. Ginkgo is now grown on plantations to supply the ever-increasing demand for this beautiful and useful tree.

POSSIBLE USES: Ginkgo leaf has been the subject of extensive modern clinical research in Europe. Its most striking clinical effect is its ability to dilate blood vessels and improve circulation and vascular integrity in the head, heart, and extremities. Reduced circulation to the head is responsible for many of the mental and neurologic symptoms of aging, including memory loss, depression, and impaired hearing. Double-blind clinical trials—considered the most reliable study method of scientific research—have shown that ginkgo can help these conditions when they are due to impaired circulation. Ginkgo also has other actions on the brain, including strengthening the vessels and promoting the action of neurotransmitters, chemical compounds responsible for the transmission of nerve impulses between brain and other nerve cells.

Because it increases circulation in the heart and limbs, ginkgo may be useful for ischemic heart disease or intermittent claudication, conditions that can occur when blood flow to the muscles is reduced because atherosclerosis has narrowed the arteries. Ginkgo dilates the clogged arteries and allows more blood flow to the muscles. Ginkgo also thins the blood, reducing its tendency to clot, another benefit in atherosclerotic disease.

Constituents in ginkgo are also potent antioxidants with anti-inflammatory effects. A common current scientific theory attributes many of the signs of aging and chronic disease to the oxidation of cell membranes by substances called free radicals. These may arise from pollutants in the atmosphere or from the normal internal production of metabolic substances. Antioxidant vitamins and other substances, including ginkgo, are currently being investigated for their ability to counter inflammation and destruction of or damage to cells from oxidation.

POSSIBLE SIDE EFFECTS: Ginkgo promotes circulation in the head and could possibly worsen congestive headaches in those who are prone to them. Because ginkgo inhibits platelets from grouping, it may cause problems for people with clotting disorders or those who take blood thinning medications. Large quantities of ginkgo may cause irritability, restlessness, diarrhea, and nausea and vomiting.

PRECAUTIONS AND WARNINGS: For most people, ginkgo is considered safe in recommended doses. Ginkgo extract is a prescription drug in Europe because most of the conditions that it benefits are not suitable for self-medication. If you have memory loss, depression, or the symptoms of atherosclerosis, you should see a physician for a diagnosis. Patients with a diagnosis of benign senility may safely take ginkgo.

If you have had a stroke or think you are prone to them for any reason, don't take ginkgo without your physician's permission. Although it thins the blood, which could be beneficial for one kind of stroke, it also increases circulation to the brain, which could promote another kind.

PART USED: Leaf extract (The seed or nut is used in Chinese medicine but for entirely different purposes. The nuts are also used in Oriental cooking.)

PREPARATION AND DOSAGE: Ginkgo leaf extract is available in teas, tinctures, extracts, and capsules; however, only the capsules, which are standardized for their flavonoid content, have the substances that may cause side effects removed. The unstandardized forms frequently cause headache and gastrointestinal upset. Look for capsules with 24 percent flavonoid content. To receive the same benefits attributed to standardized ginkgo capsules, you would have to consume large quantities of tincture, tea, or powder. These quantities would place you at greater risk for side effects, such as serious headaches and gastrointestinal upset.

You may safely take 2 to 6 ginkgo capsules a day. Begin with 3 capsules and increase after two months if no effects are noted.

GINSENG, AMERICAN AND ASIAN

Panax quinquefolius, Panax ginseng
Family: Araliaceae

So POPULAR IS THIS herb that more than 50,000 people are employed worldwide in the ginseng industry. Rather than addressing specific conditions, ginseng is used to treat underlying weakness that can lead to a variety of conditions. For example, among its many uses, ginseng is recommended for people who are frequently fatigued, weak, stressed, and affected by repeated colds and flu.

The enthusiasm over ginseng began thousands of years ago in China where *Panax ginseng* grows. So valued was China's native species, the plant was overharvested from the wild, causing scarcity and increased demand. A mature, cultivated woods-grown root of *P. ginseng* will sometimes fetch $1,000 or more. A mature, *wild* woods-grown root of *P. ginseng* will sometimes fetch $200,000 or more! When a similar species, *P. quinquefolius*, was noted in the early American colonies, tons of the plant were immediately dug and exported to China. Many American pioneers made their living digging ginseng roots from moist woodlands. As a result, ginseng has become rare in its natural habitat in the United States as well. Ginseng is now cultivated in forests or under vast shading tarps.

Many people believe the cultivated ginseng has slightly different properties than the natural wild specimens. The Asian species is said to be a superior medicine than the American species, but the two species have slightly different applications. The Asian *P. ginseng* is said to be a yang tonic, or more warming, while the American *P. quinquefolius* is said to be a yin tonic, or more cooling. Both the *ginseng* and the *quinquefolius* species are qi tonics, or agents capable of strengthening qi, our vital life force.

In traditional Chinese medicine, our vital qi is composed of two opposing forces, yin and yang. Yin and yang are dualistic opposites that churn and cycle in all life and, indeed, all matter. The yang aspect of the life forces is the bright, hot, masculine, external, dispersive, dynamic pole. The yin aspect is the dark, moist, feminine, internal, contracted, mysterious pole. All people, all plants, all matter, yes, even all diseases, have their yin and yang aspects. Traditional Chinese medicine is very sophisticated in its observation of this phenomena, thus all botanical therapies are fine-tuned accordingly. *P. ginseng*, for example, might be recommended to warm and stimulate someone who is weak and cold from nervous exhaustion. *P. quinquefolius,* on the other hand, is best for someone who is hot, stimulated, and restless from nervous exhaustion and feverish wasting disease. It is good for someone experiencing a lot of stress (and subsequent insomnia). American ginseng is used in China to recuperate from fever and the feeling of fatigue associated with summer heat.

POSSIBLE USES: Asian ginseng is used as a general tonic by modern Western herbalists as well as by traditional Chinese practitioners. It is thought to gently stimulate and strengthen the central nervous system in cases of fatigue, physical exertion, weakness from disease and injury, and prolonged emotional stress. Its most widespread use is among the elderly. It is reported to help control diabetes, improve blood pressure and heart action, and reduce mental confusion, headaches, and weakness among the elderly. Asian ginseng's affinity for the nervous system and its ability to promote relaxation make it useful for stress-related conditions such as insomnia and anxiety. Serious athletes may benefit from the use of Asian ginseng with improved stamina and endurance. The Asian species is also reported to be a sexual tonic and aphrodisiac useful in maintaining the reproductive organs and sexual desire into old age.

Animal and human studies have shown Asian ginseng possibly reduces the occurrence of cancer: Ginseng preparations increase production of immune cells, which may boost immune function.

Ginseng contains many complex saponins referred to as ginsenosides. Ginsenosides have been studied extensively and found to have numerous complex actions, including the following: They stimulate bone marrow production, stimulate the immune system, inhibit tumor growth, balance blood sugar, stabilize blood pressure, and detoxify the liver, among many other tonic effects. Ginseng also contains numerous other constituents; yet no one constituent has been identified as the most active. In fact, many of the individual constituents have been shown to have opposite actions. Like all plant medicine, the activity is due to the sum total of all the substances.

POSSIBLE SIDE EFFECTS: The Chinese consider the Asian species *P. ginseng* a yang tonic, so it is not used in those who have what traditional Chinese medicine refers to as yang excess, or excess heat. This means that people who are warm or red in the face or have high blood pressure or rapid heartbeat should not use Asian ginseng. American ginseng is much better suited for this type of person. But conversely, American ginseng should not be used in those who are cold or pale or those with a slow heartbeat. Possible side effects of Asian ginseng use include, curiously, some of the symptoms it is prescribed for: hypertension, insomnia, nervousness, and irritability. Acne and diarrhea are occasionally reported also. Due to potential hormonal activity, Asian ginseng can promote menstrual changes and breast tenderness on occasion. The side effects caused by ginseng resolve quickly once the herb is discontinued. Seek advice from an herbalist or naturopathic physician who can determine if ginseng is appropriate for you and, if so, recommend an appropriate dose.

PRECAUTIONS AND WARNINGS: Ginseng is one of the better researched plants, and no serious toxicity has ever been reported. Due to hormonal activity, however, ginseng should be avoided during pregnancy. Some cases of hypertension are aggravated by ginseng while others are improved; consult an herbalist or naturopathic physician for the use of ginseng in hypertension.

PART USED: Root (Cultivated roots are grown for four to six years to bring them to market weight. Wild roots of similar weight are often 50 to 100 years of age and thought to be superior.)

PREPARATION AND DOSAGE: Due to the widespread and long-term use of ginseng, ways to prepare, ingest, and dose it abound, and no single recommendation can be made. Ginseng is dried for teas, powdered and encapsulated, candied, tinctured, and made into concentrates and syrups. Use from 2 to 8 grams of the dried root per day. This amount is equivalent to 4 to 6 capsules or 1 tablespoon of tincture each day. Many herbalists recommend using ginseng in an on-and-off pattern of several weeks on, and a week or two off. Not only does ginseng seem more effective this way, but this regimen reduces the likelihood of overstimulation and side effects.

GOLDENSEAL

Hydrastis canadensis
Family: Ranunculaceae

❦

THE ROOT OF THIS LOW-GROWING woodland plant is cultivated in the fall as an impor-
tant antimicrobial agent. So
extensive has its use been, in fact,
that overharvesting
has all but wiped out
wild goldenseal. To
protect this popular
herb from extinction, you
should never dig up wild
goldenseal plants or buy
from anyone who does. This
botanical is now farmed in
woodland settings to meet
the great market demand
without further endangering goldenseal in its natural setting. And the demand is indeed great:
More than 150,000 pounds of goldenseal is consumed annually in America alone!

POSSIBLE USES: Goldenseal is so valued because
it is a strong antimicrobial and a mild anti-
inflammatory. Its astringent properties make it
useful to treat conditions of the throat, stomach,
and vagina when these tissues are inflamed,
swollen, or infected. The yellow-pigmented powder also makes a good antiseptic skin wash for

wounds and for internal skin surfaces, such as in the vagina and ear canal. Goldenseal eye washes are useful for simple conjunctivitis.

An anti-inflammatory and antimicrobial astringent, goldenseal is particularly effective on the digestive system—from the oral mucosa to the intestinal tract. It is helpful for canker sores in the mouth and as a mouth rinse for infected gums. For sore throats, goldenseal works well combined with echinacea and myrrh. Gargling with goldenseal is effective, too; extended surface contact with the infected area is ideal treatment. Irritable bowel diseases also benefit from the use of goldenseal when there is diarrhea and excessive intestinal activity and secretions. For general debility of the stomach and digestion such as chronic gas, indigestion, and difficulty with absorption of nutrients, herbalists recommend a combination of equal parts goldenseal and cayenne pepper in tincture or capsules before meals on a regular basis. Goldenseal has been found useful in treating the many types of diarrhea commonly seen in AIDS patients. Weakened immune function makes people susceptible to intestinal and other infections; goldenseal can help prevent and treat these infections.

Goldenseal has been found to be effective against a number of disease-causing organisms, including *Staphylococcus*, *Streptococcus*, and *Chlamydia* species and many others. Berberine and related alkaloids in goldenseal have been credited with its

SORE THROAT REMEDY

Combine equal parts of goldenseal, echinacea, and myrrh tinctures. Gargle then swallow. This formula tastes awful, but it's well worth the grimacing. For best results, take ¼ to ½ teaspoon four to eight times a day as soon as sore throat begins. Reduce to three or four times a day in two or three days. Note: If the sore throat persists, see a physician.

antimicrobial effects. Berberine may be responsible for the increased white blood cell activity associated with goldenseal use, as well as its promotion of blood flow in the liver and spleen. Promoting circulation in these organs enhances their general function. Berberine has been used recently in China to combat the depression of the white blood cell count that commonly follows chemotherapy and radiation therapy for cancer. Both human and animal studies suggest berberine may have potential in the treatment of brain tumors and skin cancers. Since goldenseal acts as an astringent to mucosal tissues, it has been recommended to treat oral cancers as well as abnormal cells in the cervix (cervical dysplasia) and cervical cancer. The astringent and immune-stimulating action of goldenseal seems to heal inflamed cells and eliminate abnormal cells.

Goldenseal has the curious reputation as an herb people take before undergoing a drug test to ensure they pass. There is no logical basis for this; herbalist author and photographer Steven Foster cleared up this rumor when he pointed out it stemmed from the plot of a fictional murder mystery written by a prominent herbalist, John Uri Lloyd, almost a century ago.

POSSIBLE SIDE EFFECTS: Goldenseal is considered quite safe but, due to its alkaloid content, should be avoided during pregnancy. Researchers and herbalists disagree, however, about whether goldenseal can impair the beneficial bacteria of our digestive tracts the way that pharmaceutical antibiotics can. Not all bacteria is harmful; our bodies need some types of bacteria to assist in digestion, for example. So if you are one of the rare individuals who needs to use goldenseal long-term, you should supplement your diet with *Lactobacillus acidophilus* bacterial strains, such as those found in active-culture yogurt, to replenish the body's supply of beneficial bacteria.

PRECAUTIONS AND WARNINGS: Because of the overharvesting of goldenseal, many herbalists recommend using goldenseal only occasionally, recommending use of other antimicrobial herbs, such as Oregon grape, thyme, or garlic in its place whenever possible. Be aware that goldenseal is also used as a yellow dye, so medicinal tinctures and teas will permanently stain clothing. Don't worry, though: Topical applications won't stain your skin or your eyes, if you use the eyewash.

PART USED: Root

PREPARATION AND DOSAGE: Goldenseal's extremely bitter taste makes it more appropriate for tinctures and capsules rather than teas.

Tincture: Use ¼ to ½ teaspoon every one to two hours in adults with an acute sore throat or intestinal infection. When treating infections with herbal preparations, it is usually best to take a dose fairly frequently at the onset of symptoms, and reduce the frequency in the following days as symptoms improve.

Capsules: Take 1 or 2 capsules every two to four hours when an infection first begins, and then reduce the frequency over several days' time. This botanical is fine for children and the elderly, but they require a lower dosage. Be sure to check with an herbalist for the appropriate dosage.

HAWTHORN

Crataegus laevigata
Family: Rosaceae

❀

*L*IKE MANY MEMBERS of the rose family, the hawthorn bears lovely, fragrant flowers; brightly pigmented fall berries high in vitamin C; and a few thorns. The hawthorn has been a cherished plant for centuries and is mentioned in many of the old European herbals. A popular ornamental and landscaping plant, this beautiful tree flowers in May, thus it is sometimes called the mayflower. The pilgrims that traversed the Atlantic centuries ago may have named their ship the Mayflower after the prosperous hawthorn tree.

Reverence for the hawthorn in Europe is an ancient tradition. The ancient European druids included the hawthorn with the sacred oak and the ash in a trio of trees with special powers. Europeans often left offerings of food at the base of hawthorn trees for the fairies, or little folk. Superstitions of harm coming to those who chopped down or pruned a hawthorn prevented many from tampering with the sacred tree in any way. Many people would not even bring the spring flowers inside, lest they upset the little folk.

POSSIBLE USES: Hawthorn is an important botanical cardiotonic (capable of producing and restoring the normal tone of the heart), and medications are made from the flowers and, especially, berries of the hawthorn tree. Hawthorn's many chemical constituents include the flavonoids anthocyanidins and proanthocyanidins, which reduce blood vessel sensitivity to and damage from oxidizing agents. Various chemicals in our environment—pollutants, smoke, and chemicals in food—can bind to and damage the lining of blood vessels. Hawthorn improves the integrity of veins and arteries, enhancing circulation and nutrition to the heart, thus improving the function of the heart muscle itself. This action makes it useful for cases of angina (chest pain), atherosclerosis (a buildup of fat on the inside of artery walls), weakness and enlargement of the heart, high and low blood pressure, and elevated cholesterol levels. Hawthorn may also help control arrhythmias and palpitations. Early American Eclectic physicians suggested that hawthorn be used for valvular problems of the heart, especially when accompanied by a fast heart rate and nervousness. Modern herbalists continue to use hawthorn for such complaints.

POSSIBLE SIDE EFFECTS: Hawthorn is considered quite safe, and it may be used long-term under supervision of a healthcare professional.

WARNINGS AND PRECAUTIONS: There are no known toxicities; however, hawthorn preparations can potentiate (intensify) the action of some medications, making a lesser dosage required. Consult an herbalist or physician regarding the use of hawthorn, particularly with heart medications.

PART USED: Ripe berries and flowers

PREPARATION AND DOSAGE: The flowers are tinctured in the spring and the berries tinctured in the fall and the resulting liquids mixed together to provide the full complement of active chemical constituents. The berries are quite tasty, so those with heart disease or blood pressure problems can snack on the berries or use them to prepare medicinal foods such as hawthorn berry jam.

Tincture: Take 20 to 30 drops three times a day.

❀ ❀ ❀

Hawthorn Berry Jam

1 pound fresh, ripe hawthorn berries (around 3 cups)	8 cups water
	Honey
	Juice of 1 lemon
1 pound fresh apples, chopped (about 2 medium)	

Simmer the fruit in the water until soft and thick and much of the water has evaporated. Place in a jelly bag and leave to drip in a bowl overnight to remove the hawthorn pits and other large particles. Measure the strained liquid and add an equal amount of honey. Simmer the mixture, skimming any scum that forms on the top. Add the juice of 1 lemon, stir, and pour into clean jars. Refrigerate. Use syrup on pancakes, desserts, and fresh fruit and as a sweetener in teas.

HOPS

Humulus lupulus
Family: Moraceae

POSSIBLE USES: Hops are perhaps best known for their use as a bitter agent in brewing beer. But hops are also a nerve sedative and hormonal agent. Because they promote stomach secretions, bitter herbs are good digestive tonics. The bitter principles in hops are particularly useful for indigestion aggravated by stress or insufficient stomach acid and for gassiness and sour burping. Research has shown that hops may also help the body metabolize natural toxins such as those produced by bacteria.

Hops contain plant estrogens, and women who harvest hop flowers for an extended time sometimes develop menstrual-cycle abnormalities. Its estrogenic constituents make this plant useful to treat menopausal complaints, such as insomnia and hot flashes.

You may also use hops for anxiety and nervous complaints or for indigestion and cramps resulting from anxiety. Use the tincture or tea before bed if you experience insomnia.

POSSIBLE SIDE EFFECTS: Nausea and stomach upset from stimulation of digestive secretions occurs occasionally. Menstrual-cycle irregularities occur rarely. A small number of people who try hops for nervousness and insomnia find their symptoms worsen, or they experience a dull headache. If this happens to you and the symptoms do not abate, stop taking hops. Try a lower dose several weeks later.

PRECAUTIONS AND WARNINGS: Hops are considered safe for occasional use as a beverage or medication.

PART USED: Strobiles (plain flowers) harvested during the summer

PREPARATION AND DOSAGE: Hops are used in beers, teas, tinctures, and capsules. To make tea, steep 1 to 2 tablespoons of hops flowers in a cup of hot water for 15 minutes.

For digestive stimulation: Take 1 to 2 hops capsules or a dropper full (¼ teaspoon) of tincture 20 minutes before meals.

For anxiety: Drink 2 to 3 cups of tea made from hops and skullcap throughout the day.

For insomnia caused by nerves or stomach upset: Take 2 or 3 hops capsules or 1 to 2 teaspoons of tincture half an hour before bed.

HORSERADISH

Armoracia rusticana
Family: Brassicaceae

POSSIBLE USES: Have you ever bitten into a roast beef sandwich and thought your nose was on fire? The sandwich probably contained horseradish. Even a tiny taste of this potent condiment seems to go straight to your nose. Whether on a sandwich or in a herbal preparation, horseradish clears sinuses, increases facial circulation, and promotes expulsion of mucus.

Horseradish is helpful for sinus infections because it encourages your body to get rid of mucus. One way a sinus infection starts is with the accumulation of thick mucus in the sinuses: Stagnant mucus is the perfect breeding ground for bacteria to multiply and cause a painful infection. Horseradish can help thin and move out older, thicker mucus accumulations. If you are prone to developing sinus infections, try taking horseradish the minute you feel a cold coming on. Herbalists also recommend horseradish for common colds, influenza, and lung congestion. Incidentally, don't view the increase of mucus production after horseradish therapy as a sign your cold is worsening. The free-flowing mucus is a positive sign that your body is ridding itself of wastes.

Horseradish has a mild natural antibiotic effect and it stimulates urine production. Thus, it has been used for urinary infections.

Occasionally, horseradish is used topically to alleviate the pain of arthritis and nerve irritation. Horseradish also has been used as a poultice to treat infected wounds.

POSSIBLE SIDE EFFECTS: Pain in the head, especially behind the root of the nose, is a common but brief side effect. Large, repetitive doses of horseradish may cause stomach upset and even vomiting in some people. Rashes and inflammation may follow topical use. If you experience gastrointestinal distress after eating other sulfur-containing cruciferous vegetables, such as cabbage or broccoli, you may not want to use horseradish. You may experience an upset stomach even if the amount you consume is neither particularly large nor repetitive.

PRECAUTIONS AND WARNINGS: Avoid prolonged exposure to horseradish's volatile fumes, which may irritate the lungs and cause a burning sensation.

PART USED: Root

PREPARATION AND DOSAGE: Horseradish root keeps for several months in a resealable plastic bag in the refrigerator. (Fresh root is superior as a medicine, but commercially prepared horseradish will do in a pinch.) Grate the horseradish in a food processor or blender. Add honey or sugar and vinegar to taste (about 2 tablespoons honey or sugar and 1 tablespoon vinegar per cup of horseradish). If you can tolerate its flavor, spread ¼ teaspoon of prepared horseradish on a cracker and eat it. Or stir the horseradish in a sip of warm water with a little honey.

You can make a horseradish poultice to treat a wound, or soak a cloth in horseradish tea and apply the cloth to the wound. Discontinue if the skin reddens or causes irritation or a rash.

Tincture: Take ¼ to ½ teaspoon of horseradish tincture at a time, straight or in warm water, every hour or so to clear head congestion.

Tea: Steep 1 teaspoon fresh grated horseradish in hot water and sip for congestion. Add honey, lemon, or other herbs to balance the flavor.

🌺 🌺 🌺

Horseradish-Cranberry Holiday Relish

1 cup freshly grated horseradish root	2 Tbsp vinegar
	¼ cup honey
2 cups organic cranberries	½ cup sour cream

Blend ingredients in a blender or food processor to create a beautiful pink condiment that will get your taste buds' attention, as well as treat your winter colds.

HORSETAIL

Equisetum arvense
Family: Equisetaceae

❦

T HE LATIN ROOT *Equis* and common name horsetail refer to this primitive plant's thin, branchlike leaves, which resemble the coarse hair of a horse's tail. The other common name, scouring rush, derives from the tough plant's use as a natural scouring pad for pots and pans.

POSSIBLE USES: Horsetail is used medicinally to treat bladder infections and bladder weakness. Adults who experience occasional nocturnal incontinence (bed-wetting) may benefit from using horsetail. The herb relieves a persistent urge to urinate.

Horsetail is classified as a diuretic, but sources differ as to its strength. Horsetail tea or tincture may help people who experience edema (fluid buildup) in the legs caused by such conditions as rheumatoid arthritis and circulatory problems.

Because it contains silica and minerals, horsetail often is used to strengthen bone, hair, and fingernails—parts of the body that require high mineral levels. You may drink horsetail tea every day, for no longer than a month, if you've broken a bone.

Horsetail also may be used by those who have wounds that do not heal well.

POSSIBLE SIDE EFFECTS: Kidney irritation could occur with long-term, repetitive, and frequent use. Limit its use to one month.

PRECAUTIONS AND WARNINGS: Avoid horsetail if you have high blood pressure or a family history of silica kidney stones. Horsetail may make breast milk less palatable to nursing infants. Ask herb suppliers where they gathered their horsetail. Make sure it doesn't come from roadsides or other possibly polluted environments. Horsetail is known to concentrate heavy metals and other toxins in its leaves.

PART USED: Entire plant

PREPARATION AND DOSAGE: Gather young shoots early in the spring and eat like asparagus, or dry and tincture. Don't gather horsetail late in the season because its silica levels will be too high. For chronic conditions, such as osteoporosis and other bone-thinning diseases, take horsetail for a week, and abstain for a week or two before resuming use.

Tincture: Most people can tolerate 30 to 60 drops of horsetail tincture two to five times a day. But don't take horsetail for longer than a month.

Tea: Boil 1 tablespoon of horsetail per cup of water; drink 2 to 4 cups a day for a week.

JUNIPER

Juniperus communis
Family: Cupressaceae

POSSIBLE USES: With their warming, stimulating, and disinfecting actions, juniper berries have many medicinal uses. They have an antiseptic effect and are often used in cases of chronic and repeated urinary tract infection between flare-ups not, however, for acute cases of bladder infection.

Juniper stimulates urinary passages, so the kidneys move fluids faster. This is helpful if your kidneys are working sluggishly (such as with renal insufficiency), and urine is not flowing freely. But such stimulation would be disastrous if you had a kidney infection. Juniper must be used judiciously, starting with small, cautious dosages. Use it also for prolapse and weakness of the bladder or urethra. Because juniper is indicated for chronic conditions associated with debility and lack of tone in the tissues, it is most used for treating older people or those with chronic diseases. Both the aging process and prolonged disease are associated with loss of tone in tissues and organs. Since juniper is stimulating, it is useful in these situations.

Juniper berries also are recommended for joint pain, gout, rheumatoid arthritis, and nerve, muscle, and tendon disorders. The plant is used internally and topically for such complaints in small doses over several weeks. Take it for a week; then abstain for two.

Juniper is valuable for respiratory infections and congestion because the essential oil in its berries opens bronchial passages and helps to expel mucus. Juniper's essential oils have been used topically for coughs and lung congestion. Its tars and resins have been isolated and used topically to treat psoriasis and other stubborn skin conditions. In both topical therapies, juniper has a warming, stimulating, and irritating action.

Juniper also is considered a uterine stimulant, occasionally used by herbalists to improve uterine tone and late or slow-starting menstrual periods. Juniper's essential oils also relieve gas in the digestive system and increase stomach acid when insufficient. Some hydrochloric acid in the stomach is required to digest food; insufficient acid leads to incomplete digestion, gassiness, and bloating.

POSSIBLE SIDE EFFECTS: Irritation of the urinary passages may occur if juniper is not used properly. Its use requires knowledge and caution. Because juniper increases stomach acid, it may upset some people's stomachs.

PRECAUTIONS AND WARNINGS: Avoid juniper during pregnancy. Large doses of juniper such as 5 to 6 cups of strong tea may cause vomiting, diarrhea, and increased urine flow. Such dosages taken day after day may poison the kidneys and cause convulsions. Juniper should not be used by anyone with acute kidney inflammation. Juniper is better suited for urinary atony such as a weak or prolapsed bladder, and minor infections that do not involve the kidneys.

Use juniper only for a month or so, then abstain for a week or more before using the herb again.

PART USED: Dark blue (ripe) cones, commonly referred to as berries

PREPARATION AND DOSAGE: Juniper berries may be tinctured or stored whole. Because juniper's volatile oils may irritate and stimulate, keep the dosage low. When making juniper tea, short, hot infusions of just five to eight minutes are best to preserve the volatile oils. Steep about 20 berries per cup of hot water. Steep in a covered container to preserve the oils.

Tea: Limit consumption to 1 or 2 cups in a day, and do not use longer than two months.

Tincture: Take 10 to 30 drops at a time, no more than four times a day. Limit use to four to six weeks. Start with a low dosage and work upward if needed.

LAVENDER

Lavandula angustifolia
Family: Labiatae

❧

POSSIBLE USES: Lavender has been cherished for centuries for its sweet, relaxing perfume. The word lavender comes from the Latin root *lavare*, meaning to wash, since lavender was frequently used in soaps and hair rinses.

Besides its importance as a fragrance, lavender is considered calming to nervous tension. Lavender oil is sometimes rubbed into the temples for head pain, put into the bath water for an anxiety-reducing bath, or put on a cotton ball and placed inside a pillowcase to treat insomnia. Lavender flowers are added to tea formulas for a pleasing, soothing aroma as well as for a calming effect on the psyche; the tea is sipped throughout the day to ease nervous tension. Lavender has a mildly sedating action and is also a weak antispasmodic for muscular tension.

Lavender may also alleviate gas and bloating in intestines as most herbs high in volatile oils are reported to do. One of lavender's volatile oils, linalool, has been found to relax the bronchial passages, reducing inflammatory and allergic reactions. Lavender is sometimes included in asthma,

USING LAVENDER ESSENTIAL OIL

Add lavender essential oil to the last few minutes of the rinse cycle in your washing machine when laundering your sheets, towels, and lingerie. Soak a cotton ball with lavender essential oil, tie it inside a small piece of fabric, and tuck it in your pillowcase or put it inside your dresser drawers. Place a drop or two of lavender oil on a cool lightbulb of the lamp near your bed, for a calming effect when you read in bed.

Do not use concentrated essential oils internally. Do not use in doses larger than a drop or two and always dilute with water or an oil such as almond or any vegetable oil. Putting a drop of some oils on the skin or tongue can cause burns with blisters.

cough, and other respiratory formulas. Linalool is also credited as an expectorant and antiseptic.

POSSIBLE SIDE EFFECTS: Some people dislike the smell of lavender and find it nauseating or irritating to the nose.

PRECAUTIONS AND WARNINGS: Do not take lavender in large or therapeutic doses during pregnancy.

PART USED: Flowers, harvested in the initial stages of flowering

PREPARATION AND DOSAGE: Lavender is commonly added to soaps, perfumes, powders, and potpourri blends. Enormous quantities of lavender are steam-distilled to prepare the concentrated essential oils, which are used in the perfume and cosmetic industry and are available in pure form in health food stores and perfume shops. The essential oils may be used topically (always dilute before applying the essential oil to the skin) and in the practice of aromatherapy (the use of strong smelling substances to elicit a medicinal effect).

You can add dried lavender flowers to tea formulas. Briefly steep 1 teaspoon to 1 tablespoon of flowers per cup of hot water. When infusing lavender, use a lid to prevent the essential oils from escaping into the air.

LEMON BALM

Melissa officinalis
Family: Labiatae

POSSIBLE USES: Crush a single lemon balm leaf and rub it on your skin or clothing and it smells lemony for hours. The smell of the fresh plant is described as sharp, vibrant, and stimulating, and lemon balm is used medicinally to sharpen and stimulate the senses. Lemon balm is classified as a stimulating nervine, or nerve tonic, and though it has a soothing effect on the nervous system and alleviates anxiety, it is not a simple sedative. Lemon balm is particularly indicated for nervous problems that have arisen from longstanding worry and stress, and anxiety accompanied by headache, sluggishness, confusion, depression, and exhaustion.

Lemon balm is also credited with an antiviral effect, and it seems particularly effective against the herpes virus. Lemon balm alleviates stomach gas and cramps and has a general antispasmodic effect on the stomach and intestines. It also relaxes the blood vessels, helping to reduce blood pressure.

POSSIBLE SIDE EFFECTS: None commonly reported

PRECAUTIONS AND WARNINGS: None cited; lemon balm is considered safe even for infants, the elderly, and the infirm.

PART USED: Leaves

PREPARATION AND DOSAGE: To make tea, use a handful of crushed, fresh leaves per teapot. Add a drop or two of concentrated essential oil of lemon balm to tinctures and teas. Inhale lemon balm oil in small amounts for aromatherapy. To treat herpes lesions of the lips, rub diluted essential oil on the lesions.

❧ ❧ ❧

Lemon Balm Sorbet

2 large apples, chopped	2 cups water
Leaves from 6 lemon balm sprigs	1 cup honey
	Juice of 2 lemons

Purée apples and lemon balm in a blender or food processor. Transfer purée to a saucepan. Add water and honey. Simmer over low heat until thick and bubbly. Strain. Add lemon juice, stir briskly, and cool. Place mixture in an ice cream maker and freeze. If you don't have an ice cream maker, freeze, then blend the mixture just before serving. Garnish with fresh lemon balm sprigs, and serve with scones or tea biscuits.

LICORICE
Glycyrrhiza glabra
Family: Leguminosae

❧

WHEN YOU WERE a child, did you like the black jelly beans best? Then you would love drinking licorice tea or chewing on a licorice root. At one time black licorice and other candy was flavored with licorice roots. Although today licorice candy usually derives its distinctive taste from anise oil, the root is still prized as a flavoring agent and a medicine and is used widely in the food and health industries. Licorice may be found in the wild, but large crops are farmed to meet a demand for this important botanical.

POSSIBLE USES: Licorice is used to treat a vast array of illnesses. In China, licorice is considered a great balancing or harmonizing agent and is added to numerous herbal formulas. It is used to soothe coughs and reduce inflammation, soothe and heal ulcers and stomach inflammation, control blood sugar, and balance hormones. Licorice is great for healing canker sores and cold sores (herpes simplex virus type I). Licorice is a potent antiviral agent and can be used to treat flu and viruses in addition to the herpesvirus. Licorice is also a strong anti-inflammatory agent and can be used to improve the flavor of other herbs. With all of these uses, it is no wonder licorice finds its way into so many therapies.

Several modern studies have demonstrated the ulcer-healing abilities of licorice. Unlike most popular ulcer medications, such as cimetidine (Tagamet), licorice does not dramatically reduce stomach acid; rather, it reduces the ability of stomach acid to damage stomach lining by encouraging digestive mucosal tissues to protect themselves from acid. Licorice enhances mucosal protection by increasing mucous-secreting cells, boosting the life of surface intestinal cells, and increasing microcirculation within the gastrointestinal tract. This improves the health of the stomach lining and reduces damage from stomach acid. One study in Ireland showed a licorice extract to be a better symptom reliever than Tagamet for a number of ulcer patients.

The remarkably sweet saponin glycoside glycyrrhizin gives licorice its characteristic flavor. (Glycyrrhizin is 60 times sweeter than sugar.) Glycyrrhizin is an anti-inflammatory, and licorice also has been used to treat inflammations of the lungs, bowels, and skin. Glycyrrhizin is one of the constituents found to prolong the length of time that cortisol, one of the adrenal hormones, circulates throughout the body. Among other actions, cortisol reduces inflammation.

Anything that prolongs the life of cortisol naturally helps to reduce inflammation. Many anti-inflammatory drugs are synthetic versions of cortisol. They control conditions such as asthma, arthritis, bowel disease, and eczema by suppressing the immune system—halting the body's ability to mount an inflammatory response. Licorice is not thought to suppress the immune system the way pharmaceutical steroids do. However, both pharmaceutical cortisones and licorice may cause the same side effects: weight gain, fluid retention, and, as a possible result, high blood pressure. Still, if you use cortisone, prednisone, or a similar steroid, you should seek the advice of a naturopathic or other knowledgeable physician to determine whether your condition may be managed another way.

POSSIBLE SIDE EFFECTS: Licorice may raise blood pressure in people with hypertension. So if you have high blood pressure, even if it is controlled with medication, avoid eating real licorice candy or using licorice as a medicine. Licorice does not tend to raise blood pressure in people who do not have high blood pressure. Licorice also may occasionally cause bloating and fluid retention, but this usually occurs only with very high doses such as more than five cups of tea per day or long-term use of lower doses, such as several months of daily consumption. Avoid licorice during pregnancy.

PART USED: Root

PREPARATION AND DOSAGE: Licorice may be purchased encapsulated, dried, and tinctured. Licorice also is processed to form elixirs and syrups. The dosages for licorice vary a great deal: Small amounts are used as a flavoring and to balance herbal formulas; large amounts—up to 3 or 4 cups per day—are used for an ulcer flare-up or irritable bowel episode. Licorice is more often used by herbalists in a formula with other herbs rather than used alone. Seek an herbalist's advice on the appropriate dosage for you.

MA HUANG, EPHEDRA

Ephedra sinica

Family: Ephedraceae

POSSIBLE USES: Ma huang is useful for treating respiratory problems and allergies—herbalists use it to open constricted bronchial airways. But it is not a safe herb to use without medical supervision. Ma huang contains an alkaloid known as ephedrine, which produces a stimulating effect, somewhat like amphetamines. Ephedrine is an ingredient found in some bronchodilators and decongestants.

Because of its stimulating effects, ma huang has found its way into numerous formulas claiming to aid in weight loss and increase energy and alertness, and even into some recreational drugs. Clearly these are inappropriate—and potentially dangerous—uses of the herb: approximately 15 deaths have been reported from chronic use or overdose of ephedra-based products. Many of these products also contain caffeine, which increases the risk of harmful effects. Simply put, the use of ma huang in weight loss products is disturbing because it has never been demonstrated to aid in long-term weight loss.

The use of ma huang in supplements purported to do everything from provide visionary experiences to producing a legal high is also sadly inappropriate. The U.S. Food and Drug Administration (FDA) continues to caution the public about the use of ma huang as a diet and energy stimulant. The FDA has, however, approved for sale ephedrine and related natural compounds as decongestants and bronchodilators.

Ma huang is sold as an herbal medication in Germany and Sweden and has been used in China for at least 5,000 years. Ma huang is useful for treating respiratory conditions, including influenza and upper respiratory infections, coughs, bronchitis, asthma, hay fever, and other airway problems caused by allergies. Ma huang is considered warming, stimulating, capable of promoting sweating, anti-inflammatory, and expectorating. When used appropriately, ma huang is effective in alleviating constriction in the chest, diminishing allergic reactivity, and reducing symptoms of asthma.

POSSIBLE SIDE EFFECTS : Because it is a stimulant, ma huang may elevate blood pressure, so avoid it if you have hypertension. Otherwise, monitor your blood pressure if you take ma huang for a long time. Ma huang also may cause heart palpitations, nervousness, trembling, sweating, and insomnia. Cardiac arrhythmias and cerebral hemorrhages have been reported in people who have taken ma huang injections.

PRECAUTIONS AND WARNINGS: Do not use ma huang unless your doctor prescribes it. Do not use it if you are pregnant, have high blood pressure, or a high fever. Do not take ma huang if you are nursing because ephedrine could contaminate your breast milk. If you have diabetes or thyroid disease, seek professional advice before using ma huang. If you take MAO inhibitors or beta-blocking drugs, stay away from ma huang products. Some sources recommend that men with enlarged prostates avoid ma huang. Do not use ma huang to lose weight, unless you are under a doctor's supervision. Do not use ma huang if you are not in good health; it may be overstimulating and dissipate your energy, rather than increase it. The elderly should not use ma huang.

PART USED: Twigs

PREPARATION AND DOSAGE: Ma huang capsules and tablets are not recommended unless prescribed by a physician or herbalist. Herbalists typically combine ma huang with other botanicals to temper its effects. Ma huang twigs are available for teas.

Tea: Boil 1 to 2 tablespoons per cup of hot water, and drink ¼ to ½ cup several times a day.

Tincture: Take ¼ to ¾ teaspoon at a time, several times a day. For a severe asthma attack, take ½ teaspoon every 15 minutes; reduce the dosage as soon as you feel better.

MARSHMALLOW

Althaea officinalis
Family: Malvaceae

❧

*T*HE MALLOW FAMILY includes the beautiful hibiscus *(Hibiscus rosa-sinensis)*, whose large, colorful blossoms grace Hawaii and other tropical environs, and hollyhocks *(Althea rosacea)*, a summer garden favorite throughout Europe and North America. All of the mallows bear lovely but short-lasting blossoms with thin, moist petals that become sticky if crushed. *Althaea* is from the Greek althino, meaning "I cure." It is so named because mallow has been used medicinally for centuries. Mallow is mentioned by Hippocrates and Culpepper in their herbals. The confection marshmallows are so named because they were originally flavored with the roots of this herb.

POSSIBLE USES: Mallow is used as a soothing demulcent to help heal skin conditions, wounds, and internal tissues. The bladder responds particularly well to mallow preparations. With the help of an herbalist, many people may improve chronic bladder infections and avoid repeated antibiotic therapy. Mallow also may be used for stomach irritation and ulcers, sore throats, coughs, and bronchitis. Mallow preparations may be used topically to treat abrasions, rashes, and inflammations.

POSSIBLE SIDE EFFECTS: None reported: Mallows are safe, soothing, and nourishing.

PART USED: Root, leaves, and flowers

PREPARATION AND DOSAGE: Chop the roots into small pieces and dry them to make teas or tinctures. If you grow your own mallow or related mallow species, dig the roots in the fall from plants two years old or more, or gather leaves or flowers in July or August when the plant is in the early stages of blooming. Use the fresh leaves and flowers in salads, too. To make mallow tea, soak 1 teaspoon to 1 tablespoon of dried root or fresh, crushed leaves or flowers per cup of cold water.

For bladder infections, sip 3 to 4 cups of mallow tea throughout the day. Antimicrobial herbs such as uva ursi, thyme, marigold, and Oregon grape are usually added to treat bacterial infections. Although you can use a tincture, teas reach the bladder and urethra faster. You will get the best results if you drink the tea as soon as symptoms develop. If you are prone to recurrent bladder infections that often require antibiotics, drink 3 to 6 cups of tea over the course of 24 hours. Decrease the dosage over several days, and then discontinue as symptoms improve.

MILK THISTLE

Silybum marianum
Family: Compositae

❧

MILK THISTLE IS AMONG the elite hand-ful of herbs that have made their way into modern hospitals. Many victims of mushroom poisoning receive milk thistle preparations to help prevent the poisons from dam-aging the liver.

POSSIBLE USES: Milk thistle is a potent antioxidant: Research has found that it significantly increases levels of glutathione, which the liver uses to detoxify and metabolize harmful sub-stances. In fact, milk thistle is used primarily to treat liver disorders, including cirrhosis and those caused by exposure to liver-damaging substances (such as alcohol and other drugs and the afore-mentioned poison mushrooms). The flavonoids in milk thistle appear to repair damaged liver cells, protect existing cells, and stimulate production of new liver cells. From a nasty hangover to a case of hepatitis, milk thistle helps the liver.

Milk thistle extracts have a preventive and thera-peutic effect when taken orally and work particu-larly well when injected intravenously. The bene-fits are demonstrated by improved symptoms and liver function tests.

POSSIBLE SIDE EFFECTS: Milk thistle is considered safe. Other than a laxative effect, no abnormalities were seen in animal toxicity trials.

PRECAUTIONS AND WARNINGS: None

PART USED: Ripe seeds

PREPARATION AND DOSAGE: Milk thistle is commonly taken in capsule, tincture, or glycerine form. Milk thistle seeds may also be roasted and ground into a nutty powder and sprinkled on food. For chronic liver toxicity or a history of chronic exposure to liver poisons such as drugs, alcohol, industrial chemicals, and other pollutants, take milk thistle daily for several months.

Capsules: Take 2 capsules two or three times a day. Double or triple the dosage for acute liver toxicity.

Tincture and glycerine: Take a dropper, or ⅛ to ¼ teaspoon of tincture, three to six times a day.

🌑 🌑 🌑
Milk Thistle-Seaweed Garnish

½ cup raw milk thistle seeds

½ cup raw sesame seeds

Dried seaweed, ground fine, or salt, to taste

In a nonstick skillet, roast milk thistle and sesame seeds for several minutes. (Don't use oil.) Stir constantly until the seeds are lightly toasted. Combine seeds with ground seaweed. Use the powder as a salty garnish on salads, pasta, rice, or wherever desired. You may also add other herbs, such as garlic, thyme, or cumin.

MOTHERWORT

Leonurus cardiaca
Family: Labiatae

POSSIBLE USES: Can you guess the medicinal actions of a plant with the name mother-wort? If you guessed that it is useful for mothers, you are right. Motherwort has been used for centuries to treat conditions of childbirth. Motherwort has the ability to act as a galactogogue, meaning it promotes a mother's milk flow. It has also been used as a uterine tonic before and after childbirth.

Motherwort is also claimed to be an emmenagogue, or an agent that promotes menstrual flow. It has been used for menopausal and menstrual complaints.

Motherwort is also a mild relaxing agent and is often used by herbalists to treat such menopausal complaints as nervousness, insomnia, heart palpitations, and rapid heart rate. The herb may help heart conditions aggravated by nervousness. In such cases, motherwort combines well with blue cohosh and ginger tinctures.

Motherwort has sometimes been referred to as a cardiotonic. Motherwort injections were recently shown to prevent the formation of blood clots, which, of course, improves blood flow and reduces the risk of heart attack, stroke, and other diseases. It is good for hypertension because it relaxes blood vessels and calms nerves. Motherwort may also correct heart palpitations that sometimes accompany thyroid disease and hypoglycemia (low blood sugar). Motherwort is also useful for headache, insomnia, and vertigo.

POSSIBLE SIDE EFFECTS: Motherwort is considered safe. However, any herb known to promote menstrual flow should be avoided by pregnant women in the first trimester.

PRECAUTIONS AND WARNINGS: Those prone to miscarriage, in particular, should avoid motherwort in pregnancy. Do not attempt to treat heart conditions without medical supervision.

PART USED: Root and flowering tops

PREPARATION AND DOSAGE: Tincture and capsules or tablets are the most common forms of motherwort medication.

Capsules: Take 1 to 4 pills per day.

Tincture: Take up to 1 tablespoon per day.

MYRRH

Commiphora molmol
Family: Burseraceae

POSSIBLE USES: So strong are the antimicrobial effects of myrrh that the ancient Egyptians relied on this plant for the process of embalming and mummification. Myrrh stimulates circulation to mucosal tissues, especially in the bronchial tract, throat, tonsils, and gums. It is useful for bleeding gums, gingivitis, tonsillitis, sore throat (including strep throat), and bronchitis. The increased blood supply helps fight infection and speed healing when you have a cold, congestion, or infection of the throat or mouth. Myrrh is also valued as an expectorant, which means it promotes the expulsion of mucus in cases of bronchitis and lung congestion. Myrrh is best for chronic conditions with pale and pus-covered tissues rather than acute, inflamed, red, and dry tissues.

Myrrh may also promote menstrual flow and is recommended when menstruation is accompanied by a heavy sensation in the pelvis. In China, myrrh is considered a "blood mover." It may alleviate menstrual cramps.

POSSIBLE SIDE EFFECTS: In small doses, myrrh is usually well tolerated. Larger doses exceeding 60 drops of tincture or frequent doses of myrrh can promote fever, burning sensations in the throat and bowels, sweating, vomiting, and diarrhea.

PRECAUTIONS AND WARNINGS: Do not exceed recommended doses or frequencies. Use myrrh to treat an infection and then discontinue use. Do not use myrrh during pregnancy.

PART USED: Stems (the gummy resin)

PREPARATION AND DOSAGE: To balance its bitter and harsh flavor, dilute myrrh with water or mix with other herbs. You can use myrrh as a mouthwash and gargle. For young children with sore throats who cannot yet gargle, place myrrh preparations in a spray bottle and squirt on the tonsils, or swab the tonsils with a cotton swab soaked in myrrh tincture. Add the concentrated essential oil of myrrh to herbal formulas for sore throats and other infections, or dilute with gold-enseal and licorice tinctures and rub on the gums with a clean fingertip. (When adding myrrh oil to tinctures, use 4 to 8 drops in a 1-ounce bottle.)

Gargle: Dissolve 1 teaspoon of myrrh tincture or ½ teaspoon of powder in 1 or 2 cups of water. Gargle and swallow the mixture. Repeat every three or four hours until you note improvement, then reduce the frequency.

Tincture: Take ½ teaspoon two or three times a day.

NETTLES

Urtica dioica
Family: Urticaceae

POSSIBLE USES: If the nettle plant has ever stung you, try not to hold a grudge because its virtues by far outweigh its offenses. Wherever nettles grow, they have been used by the local folk as a food and a medicine. Throughout early Europe, nettles were credited with nourishing and immune-stimulating properties. Nettle tea was used for intestinal weakness, diarrhea, and malnutrition—uses that persist to the present. Nettles act as a diuretic and are useful to treat kidney weakness and bladder infections. As a diuretic, nettles can help rid the body of excess fluid (edema) in persons with weakened hearts and poor circulation.

Nettles have also been used topically to treat eczema and skin rashes and soothe arthritic and rheumatic joints. In fact, the plant has been most widely studied for its value in the treatment of arthritis and gout. When uric acid, a product of protein digestion, accumulates in the joints and tissues, gout, a very painful inflammatory condition can result. One tablespoon of fresh nettle juice several times a day has been shown to help clear uric acid from the tissues and enhance its elimination from the body.

Fresh nettle preparations sting a bit, and it is this sting that seems to have a healing effect: The reddening and stinging of the skin appear to reduce the inflammatory processes of both dermatologic (such as eczema) and rheumatic conditions (such as arthritis and gout). The tiny, stinging hairs contain formic acid and a bit of histamine. (Mosquitoes and biting ants also secrete formic acid, which is responsible for the familiar stinging and itching of their bites.) Nettles are also high in anti-inflammatory flavonoids, and they contain small amounts of plant sterols. They are extremely rich in vital nutrients, including vitamin D, which is rare in plants; vitamins C and A; and minerals, including iron, calcium, phosphorus, and magnesium.

Since nettles contain numerous nourishing substances, they are used in cases of malnutrition, anemia, and rickets and as a tonic to help repair wounds and broken bones. You can cook nettles and eat them as you would steamed spinach, for their taste and appearance are similar. Nettles are a healthy and tasty addition to scrambled eggs, pasta dishes, casseroles, and soups. You can also juice nettles and combine the juice with fresh carrot, apple, or other juices to give to weak, debilitated persons, such as cancer and AIDS patients.

POSSIBLE SIDE EFFECTS: Besides the stinging rash the fresh plant can produce, side effects are uncommon. Medicinal preparations do not cause stinging or rashes—only direct contact with the living plant causes these reactions. Tingling in the mouth after drinking nettles tea occurs occasionally. Very rare allergic reactions such as dizziness and fainting have been reported.

PRECAUTIONS AND WARNINGS: Old, late-season nettles can develop hard, stony, microscopic mineral conglomerates that can irritate the kidneys and lead to swelling of urinary organs and retention of urine when used repeatedly. For this reason, young spring nettles, picked before flowering—usually in early summer—are preferred for food and medicine. Be aware that most suppliers of nettles do not pay attention to this important caution against using the older nettles. Ask about the supply of nettles your health food or herb store sells. Of course, you can grow and pick your own nettles. Otherwise, no dangers or warnings are cited commonly in modern research or literature.

PART USED: Leaves (The root is used occasionally as a hair rinse for dandruff.)

PREPARATION AND DOSAGE. Wear gloves to pick nettles in full bloom. Once the plant has been crushed, dried, cooked, or tinctured, the hairs no longer sting.

Tea: Use 1 tablespoon of dried nettle leaves per cup of hot water. Drink 2 to 4 cups per day.

Tincture: Take 1 or 2 teaspoons per day.

Juice: Drink 1 or 2 ounces per day.

❀ ❀ ❀
Nettle Pesto Pasta

Use nettles as you would greens such as steamed spinach, collards, kale, or bok choy.

3 cups small pasta
    (penne, spirals, etc.)
Fresh, young spring
    nettles, to taste
2 carrots, grated

1 large tomato, diced
1 small onion, diced
1 zucchini, sliced thin
½ cup pesto

Follow package directions to cook pasta. While the pasta is cooking, don a pair of work gloves and fill your largest pot with an inch of water and the nettles. Add remaining ingredients. Cook the nettles and vegetables in the water over medium heat until just tender. Drain the vegetables and the pasta and combine. Add pesto. Serve with bread and salad.

OATS

Avena sativa
Family: Gramineae

❧

POSSIBLE USES: Almost everyone has eaten *Avena* gruel—but you probably called it oatmeal. Oats are nourishing because they contain starches, proteins, vitamins, and minerals, and though they contain some fat, they are low in saturated fat, which makes them a healthy choice. A serving of hot oat bran cereal provides about 4 grams of dietary fiber (health professionals recommend we consume 20 to 35 grams of fiber each day). Some types of dietary fiber bind to cholesterol, and since this form of fiber is not absorbed by the body, neither is the cholesterol. A number of clinical trials have found that regular consumption of oat bran reduces blood cholesterol levels in just one month. High fiber diets may also reduce the risk of colon and rectal cancer.

Oats have been used topically to heal wounds and various skin rashes and diseases. The familiar sticky-but-smooth consistency of cooked oats is emulated in many oat products; as a result they have mucilaginous, demulcent, and soothing qualities. Soaps and various bath and body products made from oats are readily available. Oatmeal baths are wonderful for soothing dry, flaky skin or allaying itching in cases of poison oak and chicken pox. (Hint: Don't dump oatmeal right in the bath, or you'll have quite a mess. Either grind it into a fine powder or wrap it in a cloth or old nylon stocking.)

Because oats are believed to have a calming effect, herbalists recommend them to help ease the frustration and anxiety that often accompany nicotine and drug withdrawal. Oats contain the alkaloid gramine, which has been credited with mild sedative properties. Scientists have conducted clinical trials to determine whether oats may help treat drug addiction or reduce nicotine craving, but the evidence is inconclusive.

POSSIBLE SIDE EFFECTS: Although fiber helps to cleanse bowels, some people experience discomfort after suddenly increasing fiber consumption. If you have irritable bowel syndrome, your symptoms may be aggravated by abrupt addition of oat bran to your diet. But most people can tolerate gradual increases in oat bran consumption.

Some people with a food intolerance or allergy to oats may experience an eczema-like rash when handling oatmeal or oat flour. If you cannot tolerate eating oatmeal, avoid using oat-based medications.

PRECAUTIONS AND WARNINGS: As with all high fiber foods, oats should be eaten with plenty of liquid to ensure dispersal in the digestive tract. If you have celiac disease or other intolerance to gluten-containing grains, don't eat oats or take the herb as a medicine. Other than allergy or intolerance to oats, no toxicity has been noted.

PART USED: Ripe seeds (The small delicate leaves are also used medicinally but are thought to be inferior to groats for most purposes.)

PREPARATION AND DOSAGE: Oatmeal is the most common oat preparation. Whole oats, rolled oats, and oat flour are available. Oat straw and whole dried oat groats may be tinctured and used as a medicine, but oats are more commonly dried for teas. Tinctures are also available, made from the milky white secretion of the fresh oat plant. This is the form that may have a beneficial effect on nicotine and drug cravings during withdrawal.

Tea: Infuse 1 tablespoon of oats or oat straw per cup of hot water. Drink several cups a day.

Tincture: Take 1 to 2 droppers (½ to 1 teaspoon) three to four times a day.

OREGON GRAPE

Berberis aquifolium
Family: Berberidaceae
Related species: *Berberis vulgaris* (Barberry)

❧

*A*LTHOUGH OREGON GRAPE is not a true grape, it does grow in Oregon. It is indigenous to the temperate rain forests of the Pacific Northwest. The lovely shrub displays bright yellow flowers in the spring and spreads by underground stems known as rhizomes. Its blue berries are edible, though not terribly sweet, and are enjoyed by birds, bears, and small mammals. Oregon grape medicines are made from the bright yellow inner bark and young wood of the rhizomes. The bright yellow color is due to the presence of two isoquinone alkaloids, berberine and berbamine. These alkaloids are fairly strong antimicrobial agents with a broad application.

POSSIBLE USES: *Berberis* preparations are used extensively in herbal medicine for infections and to improve digestion and liver function: Oregon grape improves the flow of blood to the liver and acts as bitter tonic, stimulating the flow of bile and intestinal secretions. For these reasons, Oregon grape is often used to treat jaundice, hepatitis, poor intestinal tone and function, and general gastrointestinal dysfunction. The berberine alkaloid has been shown to benefit some patients with cirrhosis of the liver.

Oregon grape is also useful to treat colds, flu, and numerous infections. In the lab, it's been shown to kill or suppress the growth of some of the nastiest pathogens (disease-causing microbes): *Candida* and other fungi, *Staphylococcus, Streptococcus, E. coli, Entamoeba histolytica, Trichomonas vaginalis, Giardia lamblia, Vibrio cholerae,* and numerous others. Herbalists recommend it as an eyewash (since it must be highly diluted, don't try to make the eye preparations yourself), as a vaginal douche, or topically as a skin wash. Oregon grape is a nonharsh, effective alternative to antibiotics in many situations. Herbalists often use Oregon grape in place of goldenseal to ease the demand for that overharvested antimicrobial herb. Check with your naturopathic physician or herbalist regarding the treatment of infectious conditions.

POSSIBLE SIDE EFFECTS: None known

PRECAUTIONS AND WARNINGS: Because of its alkaloid content, you should avoid this herb in pregnancy. This herb is for short-term use only. In other words, use it for two to six weeks only, then stop for several weeks, resuming if necessary.

PART USED: Inner bark of the root or rhizome

PREPARATION AND DOSAGE: Oregon grape is slightly bitter, so to improve the taste of tea made from this herb, combine it with licorice, cinnamon, orange peels, or other flavorful roots and barks.

Tea: Drink 3 to 6 cups at the onset of an infection, then reduce this amount as the infection improves.

Capsules: Take 1 or 2 capsules three to four times a day.

Tincture: Take ½ teaspoon every few hours for an acute infection, decreasing the dosage as the symptoms abate.

PASSION FLOWER

Passiflora incarnata
Family: Passifloraceae

❧

POSSIBLE USES: The ancient Aztecs reportedly used passion flower as a sedative and pain reliever. Today herbalists also recommend it as a sedative and antispasmodic agent. Passion flower calms muscle tension and twitching without affecting respiratory rate or mental function, the way many pharmaceuticals do.

Passion flower has been used for anxiety, insomnia, restlessness, epilepsy, and other conditions of hyperactivity, as well as high blood pressure. Passion flower is also included in many pain formulas when discomfort is caused by muscle tension and emotional turmoil.

POSSIBLE SIDE EFFECTS: Depression of the nervous system may result in fatigue and mental fogginess if you take too much passion flower repeatedly. Start with a low dose several times a day and increase as you learn how you respond to passion flower.

PRECAUTIONS AND WARNINGS: Passion flower is generally considered nontoxic. Many herbalists prescribe 3 or 4 cups a day without any problems reported.

PART USED: Entire plant—leaf, stem, and root

PREPARATION AND DOSAGE: Passion flower is dried for teas and prepared from fresh or dry material in tinctures.

Tea: For acute stress and anxiety, drink 2 to 4 cups per day for a week; then reduce the dosage or take less often.

Tincture: For muscle tension and anxiety, take 30 to 60 drops (¼ to ½ teaspoon) of tincture from twice a day up to every two to three hours, depending on your response. Start with the smaller dose and increase amount and frequency as needed.

Capsules: Take 2 capsules two or three times a day, with a higher dose an hour before bedtime for insomnia.

PEPPERMINT

Mentha piperita
Family: Labiatae

❧

POSSIBLE USES: Peppermint is widely used as a food, flavoring, and disinfectant. As a medicine, peppermint is most well-known for its effects on the stomach and intestines. Perhaps you've tried the various tummy teas available for stomach upset. Peppermint is a tasty way to relieve gas, nausea, and stomach pain due to an irritable bowel, intestinal cramps, or indigestion. Peppermint is a carminative—an agent that dispels gas and bloating in the digestive system—and an antispasmodic capable of relieving stomach and intestinal cramps. Peppermint can be used for too much stomach acid (hyperacidity) and gastroenteritis (nausea and stomach upset that we sometimes call stomach "flu"), and it is safe for infants with colic. When treating a baby with tummy cramps, you can give a teaspoon of peppermint tea if the baby will take it, or put a cloth soaked in warm peppermint tea on the infant's belly.

Peppermint is also used topically for the cooling and relaxing effect it has on the skin. Various muscle rubs and "ices" contain peppermint oil to reduce pain, burning, and inflammation. Like other essential oils, peppermint oil is absorbed fairly well and can have a temporary pain-relieving effect on muscles and organs that are cramped and in spasm. As with all essential oils, dilute this oil before putting it directly on your skin.

Peppermint also allays itching temporarily. Rub a drop of diluted peppermint oil onto insect bites, eczema, and other itching lesions. Peppermint can help relieve some headaches, and you can rub diluted peppermint oil onto the temples or scalp for a comforting therapy.

The essential oil menthol in peppermint is credited with the analgesic, antiseptic, antispasmodic, decongestant, and cooling effect. Menthol also helps subdue many disease-producing bacteria, fungi, and viruses, but because stronger herbal antimicrobials are available, peppermint is not usually the first choice of herbalists to treat serious infections. Peppermint tea can be used as a mouthwash for babies with thrush (yeast in the mouth) or by pregnant women who wish to avoid stronger herbs and drugs.

POSSIBLE SIDE EFFECTS: Peppermint is generally recognized as safe, but people with allergies to the plant may experience headaches, stomach upset, and skin rashes.

Due to the marked antispasmodic effect, peppermint can relax the esophageal sphincter in some individuals. The esophageal sphincter is a stricture at the base of the esophagus that opens briefly to allow food to enter the stomach, and then closes again to prevent acid from the stomach from moving upward into the throat. With the sphincter relaxed, stomach acid may reflux back into the esophagus, causing inflammation and, when chronic, possibly ulceration and perforation of the esophagus. This chronic condition is called gastroesophageal reflux disease. If you have gastroesophageal reflux disease or a hiatal hernia, or you experience frequent episodes of heartburn, avoid peppermint.

PRECAUTIONS AND WARNINGS: If you have a hiatal hernia or experience reflux of stomach acid into the esophagus, peppermint could worsen the complaints. Use with caution if you have gallbladder inflammation or obstruction or advanced liver disease. Some health professionals believe peppermint may relax the bile ducts and promote bile flow. However, others have reported peppermint to be helpful in gallbladder disease, dissolving gallstones when combined with bile acid therapy.

Nursing women should consume peppermint in moderation only as it may decrease milk production. As with all essential oils, keep peppermint oil out of the eyes and open wounds.

PART USED: Leaves, gathered in the early stages of flowering

PREPARATION AND DOSAGE: Peppermint products and preparations abound. It is used commercially in toothpaste, mouthwash, breath mints, chewing tobacco substitutes, candy, and numerous other products. You can make peppermint tea with fresh leaves or commercial tea bags. Tea is the preferred choice to treat nausea and bowel complaints because the liquid comes in direct contact with the stomach and intestinal lining. Peppermint may also relieve morning sickness and is considered safe for use during pregnancy.

Tea: Drink 3 or more cups for irritable bowel, stomach cramps, or nausea.

Essential oil: Rub 1 to 10 drops of diluted oil onto the affected skin surface. Place 2 to 3 drops in a bowl of hot water and inhale the steam as a decongesting therapy.

DID YOU KNOW

Peppermint oil capsules are used to reduce the cramping that occurs with medical procedures such as sigmoidoscopies, where a physician inserts a scope in the rectum and lower bowel to visualize possible ulcers, polyps, or cancers. This procedure is understandably uncomfortable, and peppermint oil—given in specially coated capsules before the procedure—helps reduce intestinal cramping and makes such diagnostic procedures easier on the patient.

RED CLOVER
Trifolium pratense
Family: Leguminosae

❦

*H*AVE YOU EVER taken a nip of nectar from the tiny florets of this familiar meadowland plant? The bees certainly do. Clover honey is one of the most common types of honey available, and bees visit red clover throughout the summer and fall. The edible flowers are slightly sweet. You can pull the petals from the flower head and add them to salads throughout the summer. A few tiny florets are a delightful addition to a summer ice tea: Serve your summer guests a cup of iced mint tea with a lemon slice and five to ten tiny clover florets floating on top. You can also press the fresh florets into the icing on a summer birthday cake.

The raw greens of this plant are very nutritious, but like other members of the legume family (beans, peas), they are somewhat difficult to digest. The leaves are best enjoyed dried and in tea form to get the nutrients and constituents without the side effects of gas and bloating common to eating legumes.

POSSIBLE USES: Red clover's constituents are thought to stimulate the immune system. (It has been a traditional ingredient in many formulas for cancer.) Red clover has also been used to treat coughs and respiratory system congestion, since it also contains resin. Resinous substances in plants have an expectorating, warming, and antimicrobial action. Red clover also contains the blood thinning substance coumarin. Coumarin is not unique to red clover and is found in many other plants, including common grass. In fact, the pleasant sweet smell of freshly cut grass is due to the coumarin compounds. People on anticoagulant drugs such as Coumadin should be cautious of using red clover, since the blood may become too thin.

There has been much research on compounds related to coumarin of late, and many of the hormonal effects of red clover are attributed to these compounds. Here's why: When a hormone molecule is released from various organs, it travels through the bloodstream until it binds to a cell membrane, called a hormone receptor, that is able to receive it. If a compound in a plant is close enough to the shape of the body's natural hormone molecule, it may also bind to the receptor on a cell membrane. What this means is that some substances in plants produce the same effects in humans as some hormones. Coumarins in red clover are able to bind to estrogen—and possibly other—receptors. They appear to have substantial hormonal effects.

It has been noted for some time that male sheep that graze on large quantities of red clover eventually develop a diminished sperm count. (There is no evidence that red clover causes low sperm counts in human males. A human could not eat enough to affect sperm counts.) It is also common for female sheep to develop uterine fibroids. Fibroids are a noncancerous tumor; their growth within the uterine wall in humans is thought to be associated with too much estrogen in the system. It may be that the coumarins in red clover have an estrogenic effect when consumed as a staple part of the diet.

We have much to learn about coumarins, but it seems logical that they may prove useful in conditions associated with very low estrogen levels (menopause, chronic miscarriage, some cases of infertility) and should be avoided in cases of estrogen excess (uterine fibroids, endometriosis, breast cancer). Red clover has been a traditional folk therapy for infertility and chronic miscarriage, both of which can be due to insufficient estrogen.

POSSIBLE SIDE EFFECTS: On the whole, red clover is considered very safe, and little but occasional gas is noticed from drinking the tea. The mild anticoagulant effect and the hormonal effects, however, are undesirable for some individuals.

PRECAUTIONS AND WARNINGS: Those with abnormally low platelet counts, those using anticoagulants drugs, and those with clotting defects should avoid red clover preparations. Do not consume red clover before surgery or childbirth, as it may impair the ability of the blood to clot. Red clover is believed to promote the growth of uterine fibroids in sheep, but whether this is true for humans is unknown. There is also some concern that red clover may stimulate cancers that are fed by estrogen, such as some breast and uterine cancers. Until more is known, it may be best for cancer patients and those with uterine fibroids to avoid red clover.

PART USED: Flower bud and young leaves

PREPARATION AND DOSAGE:

Tea: Drink several cups of red clover tea a few times a week as a general beverage. Drink several cups daily for two to ten weeks for a medicinal effect.

Tincture: Take 2 to 4 droppers full (1 to 2 teaspoons) daily.

Red Clover Rice

Red clover blossoms
(about 100)

1 cup jasmine rice

½ cup onion, minced

½ cup peanuts, chopped

⅓ cup cabbage, chopped

⅓ cup red bell pepper,
chopped

⅓ cup carrots, grated

2 Tbsp toasted sesame
oil

2–3 Tbsp fish extract

Be sure to gather red clover from an unsprayed lawn, meadow, or pasture. Pull all of the tiny florets from the red clover flower heads.

Boil rice in 3 cups of water until soft. Strain and rinse in cold water and place in a lightly oiled skillet with onion, peanuts, cabbage, pepper, and carrots. Add sesame oil and fish extract. Cook over low heat for 15 to 20 minutes, stirring frequently. Reduce the heat to the lowest possible setting and add the red clover, stirring it in thoroughly. Let stand 5 minutes and serve as a side dish to complement steamed vegetables.

SAGE
Salvia officinalis
Family: Labiatae

❧

"**W**HY SHOULD ANYONE die who has sage in their garden?" This old saying speaks to the many conditions that can be treated with sage. The botanical name *Salvia* is from the Latin for "to save or to heal," as in the word "salvation."

POSSIBLE USES: People have been cooking with sage for thousands of years: Recipes for sage pancakes have been dated to the 5th century B.C. Like most culinary herbs, sage is thought to be a digestive aid and appetite stimulant. You can use it to reduce gas in the intestines and, because it is also antispasmodic, to relieve abdominal cramps and bloating.

Sage contains phytosterols reported to have an estrogenic as well as a cooling action. Early and modern herbals list sage as a treatment for bright red, abundant uterine bleeding and for cramps that feel worse with heat applications and better with cold applications. You may also use sage to stop breast milk production when weaning a child from breast-feeding.

The drying effect that helps dry up milk and its reported cooling action also make sage useful for treating diarrhea, colds, and excessive perspiration. It may be of value for menopausal hot flashes accompanied by profuse perspiration. Sage can dry up phlegm, and you can gargle with the tea to treat coughs and tonsil or throat infections. Sage also has been recommended as a hair rinse for dandruff, oily hair, or infections of the scalp. The herb reportedly restores color to gray or white hair.

Sage is an antioxidant and an antimicrobial agent. The volatile oils in sage kill bacteria, making the herb useful for all types of bacterial infections.

Sage may also help to lower blood sugar in people with diabetes who consume it regularly.

POSSIBLE SIDE EFFECTS: None reported

PRECAUTIONS AND WARNINGS: There have been isolated reports that the volatile oil thujone, which occurs in significant amounts in sage, may trigger seizures in people with epilepsy. Although using sage as a cooking spice is considered safe, avoid large amounts of sage as a medicinal preparation during pregnancy.

PART USED: New leaves

PREPARATION AND DOSAGE: Sage leaves may be dried for use in teas. The leaves are best infused, and most people prefer them mixed with mint, lemon grass, chamomile, or other herbs to cut the strong pungent flavor of sage.

Tea: Drink several cups of sage tea each day for a period of weeks to dry up milk flow or reduce perspiration or other secretions such as excessive mucus in the throat, nose, and sinuses. Gargling with sage tea or taking small sips throughout the day is good for throat and upper respiratory congestion.

Tincture: Take ⅛ to ½ teaspoon in a sip of water once or twice a day.

❧ ❧ ❧

Traditional Sage Stuffing

1 cup brown rice
2¼ cups soup stock, divided
1 onion, chopped
2 Tbsp sage
10 mushrooms, chopped
2 Tbsp olive or canola oil
2 carrots, grated
2 celery stalks, chopped
6 slices whole grain bread, toasted and cubed
1 cup raisins
1 cup nuts (pecans, almonds, or pine nuts), chopped

Bring rice and 2 cups of soup stock to a boil. Reduce heat, and simmer until rice is soft. While rice is cooking, heat the oil in a pan. Add the onion, mushrooms, and remaining soup stock, and cook until the onions are slightly soft. Add sage. Reduce heat to the lowest possible setting, and add carrots and celery stalks. Add the rice to the skillet along with the toast cubes. Add raisins and nuts. Stir and transfer to a baking dish. Bake for 20 to 30 minutes at 350°F. Serve as a side dish.

ST. JOHN'S WORT

Hypericum perforatum
Family: Hypericaceae

❦

ST. JOHN'S WORT is a common meadowland plant that has been used as a medicine for centuries. Early European and Slavic herbals mention it. The genus name *Hypericum* is from the Latin hyper, meaning above, and icon, meaning spirit, and the herb was, indeed, once hung over doorways to ward off evil spirits or burned to protect and sanctify an area. The species name *perforatum* refers to the many puncture-like black marks on the underside of the plant's leaves. Some sources say the plant is called St. John's wort because it blooms on St. John's Day (June 24); others say it was St. John's favorite herb; and still others note that the deep red pigment in the plant resembles the blood of the martyred saint.

POSSIBLE USES: St. John's wort has long been used medicinally as an anti-inflammatory for strains, sprains, and contusions. St. John's wort also has been used to treat muscle spasms, cramps, and the tension that often leads to muscle spasms.

The plant, especially its tiny yellow flowers, is high in hypericin and other flavonoid compounds. If you crush a flower bud between your fingers, you will release a burgundy red juice—evidence of the flavonoid hypericin. St. John's wort oils and tinctures should display this beautiful red coloring, which indicates the presence of the desired flavonoids. Bioflavonoids, in general, serve to reduce vascular fragility and inflammation. Since flavonoids improve venous wall integrity, St. John's wort is useful in treating swollen veins. St. John's wort preparations may be ingested for internal bruising and inflammation or following a traumatic injury to the external muscles and skin. The oil is also useful when applied to wounds and bruises or rubbed onto strains, sprains, or varicose veins. When rubbed onto the belly and breasts during pregnancy, the oil may also help prevent stretch marks. Topical application is also useful to treat hemorrhoids and aching, swollen veins that can occur during pregnancy.

St. John's wort is reported to relieve anxiety and tension and to act as an antidepressant. It was once thought that hypericin interferes with the body's production of a depression-related chemical called monoamine oxidase (MAO), but recent research has shed doubt on this claim. Though no one is certain how the herb works, studies have shown St. John's wort to act as a mood elevator in

AIDS patients and in depressed subjects in general. The required dosage is 3 grams of powder per day, but it must be taken weeks and sometimes several months before results are noted.

St. John's wort is useful for pelvic pain and cramping. According to the 1983 British Pharmacopoeia, St. John's wort is specifically indicated for "menopausal neuroses": Many women experience anxiety, depression, and other emotional disturbances during menopause. St. John's wort may help alleviate these symptoms.

The National Cancer Institute has conducted several studies showing that St. John's wort has potential as a cancer-fighting drug. One study showed that mice injected with the feline leukemia virus were able to fight off the infection after just a single dose of St. John's wort.

POSSIBLE SIDE EFFECTS: With long-term use, the hypericin in St. John's wort may make the skin of a few sensitive individuals more sensitive to sunlight. (This increased sensitivity to sunlight is called photophobia.) After eating large quantities of the herb, cattle developed severe sunburn and blistering.

PRECAUTIONS AND WARNINGS: None other than photophobia in very sensitive people

PART USED: Flowers and leaves picked in the early stages of flowering when the plant is highest in red pigment

PREPARATION AND DOSAGE: The fresh buds and leaves can be made into oils for topical use or dried for teas and capsules. Oils are made by soaking puréed leaves and flowers in olive oil for four to six weeks. Unlike most herbal oils, St. John's wort should be processed in direct sunlight.

Tea: Infuse 2 to 3 teaspoons per cup of hot water. Drink several cups of tea every day.

Tincture: Take ½ to ¾ teaspoon every four to eight hours.

❀ ❀ ❀

Pregnant Belly Rub

Strip the young leaves and young flower buds from St. John's wort and place in a blender with enough olive oil to cover them. Purée and transfer to a clear glass jar. Leave in the sun for three to six weeks. Shake daily. When the oil becomes a beautiful maroon color, strain and bottle. Then add one-third its amount of pure vitamin E oil, available in health food stores and mail-order catalogues. (For example, if you have 1 cup of pressed oil, add ⅓ cup vitamin E oil.) Massage this oil into the belly or breasts once or twice a day to help prevent stretch marks.

This oil is also useful for bruises, strains, and sprains. It may also promote healing and treat the pain of nerve irritation and trauma to fingertips, elbows, the tail bone, and other areas with lots of nerves.

SAW PALMETTO, SABAL

Serenoa repens
Family: Palmaceae

❧

SAW PALMETTO is a small palm tree indigenous to Florida. It is a striking, large-leaved plant that bears dark red berries the size of olives.

POSSIBLE USES: Saw palmetto has long been considered an aphrodisiac and sexual rejuvenator, although little research supports the claim. Saw palmetto does act on the sexual organs, and many herbalists value it as a treatment for impotence. The action of saw palmetto has been well studied, and the herb is popular in the treatment of prostate enlargement. Enlargement of the prostate gland affects millions of men older than 50 years of age, causing difficulty with urination and a sensation of swelling in the low pelvis or rectal area as the enlarged gland pushes on the urethra and nearby tissues. Research has shown that saw palmetto inhibits one of the active forms of testosterone in the body (dihydrotestosterone) from stimulating cellular reproduction in the prostate gland. Saw palmetto inhibits the binding of testosterone to prostate cells as well as the synthesis of testosterone. This serves to reduce multiplication of prostatic cells and reduces prostatic enlargement.

Saw palmetto is recommended to treat weakening urinary organs and the resulting incontinence that may occur in elderly people or women after menopause. It strengthens the urinary organs and has been recommended for kidney stones.

Saw palmetto has also been touted as a steroid substitute for athletes who wish to increase muscle mass, though little documentation supports this claim. Saw palmetto does affect testosterone, one of the hormones responsible for promoting muscle mass, as described above, but the precise hormonal activities on tissues other than the prostate are not yet understood. Research on other plant steroids has shown their actions to be complex and diverse. Many plant steroids, for example, enhance hormonal activity in one type of tissue and inhibit it in others. The jury is out on whether saw palmetto will pump you up, but many herbalists agree that it may benefit cases of tissue wasting, weakness, debility, weight loss, and chronic emaciating diseases. However, this may be because saw palmetto improves digestion and absorption rather than it having any hormonal effect.

POSSIBLE SIDE EFFECTS: Little information is available, but no side effects are commonly reported.

PRECAUTIONS AND WARNINGS: Men with prostate symptoms should receive a diagnosis from a physician before self-treating with saw palmetto.

PART USED: Berries

PREPARATION AND DOSAGE: Saw palmetto berries are ground into a powder and tinctured or encapsulated. For genitourinary complaints, start with the following dosages. If no improvement is noted in two to three months, you may double the dosage.

Capsules: Take 2 to 4 capsules a day.

Tincture: Take 1 to 2 teaspoons a day.

SHEPHERD'S PURSE

Capsella bursa-pastoris
Family: Cruciferae

POSSIBLE USES: Shepherd's purse is used to stop heavy bleeding and hemorrhaging, particularly from the uterus. Taken internally, shepherd's purse can reduce heavy menstrual periods, and it has been used to treat postpartum hemorrhage. Still, it is considered most effective for the treatment of chronic uterine bleeding disorders, including uterine bleeding due to the presence of a fibroid tumor. Shepherd's purse has also been used internally to treat cases of blood in the urine and bleeding from the gastrointestinal tract such as with bleeding ulcers.

An astringent agent, shepherd's purse constricts blood vessels, thereby reducing blood flow. Shepherd's purse is also thought to cause the uterine muscle to contract, which also helps reduce bleeding. There have been reports that the hemostatic action (ability to stop bleeding) of shepherd's purse is not due to the plant itself, but due to a fungus that sometimes grows on the plant. This has not been proved. There is still much to learn about shepherd's purse.

When used topically, shepherd's purse is used on lacerations and traumatic injuries to the skin to stop bleeding and promote healing. Herbalists also use the herb topically for eczema and skin rashes.

POSSIBLE SIDE EFFECTS: None commonly reported. Shepherd's purse does contain alkaloids, which can have cumulative effects in the body, so do not use this herb internally without cause.

PRECAUTIONS AND WARNINGS: Shepherd's purse has not been well researched, and its actions are not well understood. There is little reason to use shepherd's purse if you do not have bleeding problems, and you should discontinue its use as soon the problem is alleviated. Limit use to a month or two, then take a week-long break, resuming if necessary. If used for excessive menstrual bleeding, use for a few days to a week before the period and during the menstrual period—not throughout the month. Since shepherd's purse constricts the blood vessels, it is not recommended for those with high blood pressure. Pregnant and nursing women should avoid shepherd's purse.

PART USED: Flowering tops

PREPARATION AND DOSAGE: Teas and capsules of shepherd's purse are not readily available. Herbalists use shepherd's purse tincture in moderate doses of ¼ to ½ teaspoon at a time—up to a teaspoonful, three or four times a day before the menstrual period is due and during the period to reduce heavy bleeding.

SKULLCAP
Scutellaria lateriflora
Family: Labiatae
(Related species: *Scutellaria baicalensis*)

POSSIBLE USES: Skullcap is sometimes called mad dog in reference to its historical use in treating the symptoms of rabies, which can result from the bite of a rabid dog. Skullcap quiets nervous tension and eases muscle tension and spasms. It also induces sleep without strongly sedating or stupefying. Skullcap may help to lower elevated blood pressure.

Skullcap has been used for abnormally tense or twitching muscles, as with rabies, Parkinson disease, St. Vitus dance (acute chorea, a nervous system disease characterized by involuntary movements of the limbs), and epilepsy.

Skullcap has also been found to have an anti-inflammatory action. Guinea pig studies have shown that skullcap inhibits release of acetylcholine and histamine, two substances released by cells that cause inflammation.

POSSIBLE SIDE EFFECTS: Excessive use of skullcap, such as taking the tincture or capsules every ½ to 1 hour, may stimulate the central nervous system rather than sedate it. Rarely, cases of stomach cramping and diarrhea have been reported.

There have also been rare reports of skullcap causing hepatitis, but many of these cases may have resulted from mistaken use of germander, a plant that resembles skullcap.

PRECAUTIONS AND WARNINGS: None

PART USED: Leaves and the minuscule flowers

PREPARATION AND DOSAGE: Skullcap leaves and tiny flowers are dried for teas, tinctured, or powdered and encapsulated.

Tea: For severe anxiety, drink 3 to 6 cups a day for a day or two, reducing thereafter to 2 to 3 cups per day as needed. For less severe cases and long-term use, drink 1 to 3 cups a day. Prepare teas by infusing 1 tablespoon of skullcap in a cup of hot water for 15 minutes.

Tincture: Take 20 to 100 drops of tincture two to four times a day, depending on your response. Start with the low dose and increase as needed.

Capsules: Take 2 capsules two to four times a day as needed.

❧ ❧ ❧
Calming Tea

1 Tbsp skullcap	1 Tbsp chamomile
1 Tbsp passion flower	1 Tbsp lemongrass

Combine and steep in 4 cups of hot water for 15 minutes. Strain and drink throughout the day.

SLIPPERY ELM

Ulmus fulva
Family: Ulmaceae

*A*PTLY NAMED, this tree is truly slippery, but it is also elusive in another way. Once used widely by American settlers, many wild slippery elm trees have succumbed to Dutch elm disease, making the trees less 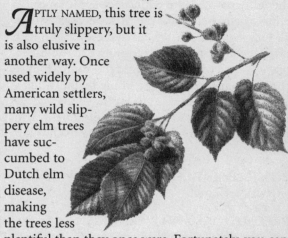 plentiful than they once were. Fortunately, you can buy slippery elm products in health food stores.

POSSIBLE USES: The species name *fulva* means tawny or pale yellow and refers to the light color of the pleasant-smelling powdered bark. Added to water, the powdered bark becomes a soothing mucilage. The mucilage moistens and soothes while the herb's tannins are astringent, making slippery elm ideal to soothe inflammations, reduce swelling, and heal damaged tissues.

Mucilage is the most abundant constituent of slippery elm bark, but the tree also contains starch, sugar, calcium, iodine, bromine, amino acids, and traces of manganese and zinc. In light of all its nourishing substances, many people eat slippery elm to soothe and nourish the body. You can stir the fluffy powder into oatmeal or apple sauce. Slippery elm helps heal internal mucosal tissues, such as the stomach, vagina, and esophagus. It is often recommended as a restorative herb for people who suffer from prolonged flu, stomach upset, chronic indigestion, and resulting malnutrition. You can use slippery elm to soothe ulcers and stomach inflammation, irritated intestines, vaginal inflammation, sore throat, coughs, and a hoarse voice.

POSSIBLE SIDE EFFECTS: Slippery elm is usually well tolerated.

PRECAUTIONS AND WARNINGS: None. Slippery elm is considered safe even for babies, the elderly, and pregnant women.

PART USED: Bark

PREPARATION AND DOSAGE: Because slippery elm does not tincture well, its bark is powdered or cut into thin strips for tea. Like all demulcents, the bark is best prepared with a long soak in cold water. The powder is most used as a healing food: Stir 2 to 3 tablespoons into juice, puréed fruit, oatmeal, or other foods. You can also mix slippery elm powder with hot water, bananas, and apple sauce to prepare an oatmeal-like gruel that can soothe an inflamed stomach or ulcer. The powder can be used to make rectal and vaginal suppositories to soothe inflammation of these tissues. In treating sore throat and coughs, try slippery elm lozenges, which you can make yourself or buy in health food stores and some pharmacies.

🌺 🌺 🌺

Slippery Elm Gruel

This recipe uses fresh apple sauce as a base. But if you're experiencing acute stomach pains and can't tolerate food, make a tea of slippery elm or whisk the powder into plain water.

Make 1 or 2 cups of fresh apple sauce, pear sauce, or nectarine purée. Add 1 cup of slippery elm powder slowly, whisking it with a fork a bit at a time. Eat as is or add raisins, maple syrup, chopped banana, or other fruit, nuts, or granola to improve the flavor.

THYME

Thymus vulgaris
Family: Labiatae

THYME HAS A LONG and varied history of both medicinal and culinary use. With its strong antibacterial actions, it has found its way into numerous formulas for respiratory, digestive, skin, and other infections. Its antiseptic properties also make it suitable as a disinfectant cleanser and an atmospheric purifier. Before the days of refrigeration, a drop of thyme volatile oil was placed in a gallon of milk to keep it from spoiling. During the plague, townspeople gathered to burn large bundles of thyme and other herbs to keep the dreaded disease from their town. Early European physicians at one time carried aromatic thyme extracts with them as they visited the sick to prevent spreading disease or becoming ill themselves. Modern studies conducted in French hospitals show that simply introducing the aroma of thyme extracts into the air helps kill germs.

POSSIBLE USES: You can drink thyme tea for relief from coughs, bronchitis, and common colds.

(Combining thyme with licorice or mint improves the flavor.) Thyme has a pronounced effect on the respiratory system; in addition to fighting infections, it dries mucous membranes and relaxes spasms of the bronchial passages. The ability of thyme to relax bronchial spasms makes it effective for coughs, bronchitis, emphysema, and asthma. Its drying effect makes it useful to reduce the abundant watering of the eyes and nose associated with hay fever and other allergies. And gargling with thyme tea can reduce swelling and pus formation in tonsillitis.

Thyme combats parasites such as hookworms and tapeworms within the digestive tract. It is also useful to treat yeast infections.

POSSIBLE SIDE EFFECTS: Side effects are uncommon with teas and tinctures. Very large dosages, such as 3 or 4 cups of thyme tea consumed all at once, may occasionally promote nausea and a sensation of warmth and perspiration. The concentrated essential oil, however, is extremely strong and irritating. When you use thyme essential oil, you must dilute it before placing it on the skin to avoid burns and inflammation.

PRECAUTIONS AND WARNINGS: Do not use essential oil of thyme topically without diluting it.

PART USED: Leaves

PREPARATION AND DOSAGE: Dilute thyme essential oil with olive or other vegetable oil and rub it into the chest and upper back to treat lung infections and coughs: Use 1 drop of thyme oil with a ½ teaspoon of olive oil; use 1 teaspoon of oil for children or those with sensitive skin. Wash your hands immediately after applying it. You can place thyme oil into a pot of steaming water and inhale the vapors to help fight infection in the nose, sinuses, and lungs. Avoid exposing your skin to steam from vigorously boiling water. Bring the water to a boil, turn the heat off, and begin the inhalation in five or ten minutes when the steam isn't too hot.

Tea: Infuse 1 teaspoon of dried or 1 tablespoon of fresh thyme in 1 cup of water. Drink 1 to 4 cups of tea per day to treat an acute respiratory infection or other type of infection.

Tincture: Take ½ teaspoon two to four times daily.

Uva Ursi

(ALSO KNOWN AS BEARBERRY, KINNIKINNICK, AND ARBUTUS)

Arctostaphylos uva-ursi
Family: Ericaceae

❀

*A*RCTO IS GREEK FOR bear and *staphylos* is Greek for a bunch of grapes, and indeed, the pink-red berries of uva ursi are a favorite of bears. Because uva ursi leaves often were mixed with tobacco and other herbs, the plant also is known as kinnikinnick, a Native American word that means smoking mixture.

POSSIBLE USES: Uva ursi is used primarily to treat urinary problems, including bladder infections. The herb is disinfecting and promotes urine flow. Uva ursi is particularly recommended to treat illnesses caused by *Escherichia coli (E. coli)*, a bacterium that commonly causes bladder and kidney infections. For kidney problems, take the herb under the care of a naturopathic physician.

Uva ursi is recommended for pelvic pain that is cramping, heavy, and dragging. The herb is particularly indicated for chronic complaints, although it should not be used for a long time. Use it for chronic irritation, pain, mucus production, and weakness of urinary organs.

POSSIBLE SIDE EFFECTS: Dosages exceeding 1½ ounces of the dried herb have poisoned some persons sensitive to this herb.

PRECAUTIONS AND WARNINGS: Avoid in pregnancy because uva ursi may stimulate the uterus. Don't take the herb for a long time because uva ursi's high tannin content may irritate your stomach. Uva ursi leaves may contain as much as 40 percent tannin when gathered late in the season. Tannins are astringent and may account for uva ursi's ability to reduce bleeding and mucus formation in the urinary passages. Be cautious about giving uva ursi to children because the herb's effects may be harsher. If you have kidney disease, take uva ursi only under the care of a physician experienced in using the herb.

PART USED: Young leaves

PREPARATION AND DOSAGE: Leaves are gathered in the spring and early summer. The leaves are evergreen and become higher in tannins in the fall. So unless you want more tannins, it is best to harvest the younger green leaves. Uva ursi is commonly used dry and tinctured.

Tincture: Take ½ to 1 teaspoon two or three times a day.

Tea: Make a decoction of the leaves to extract uva ursi's medicinal properties. Use 1 tablespoon of uva ursi leaves per 2 cups of water; boil the mixture down to 1 cup.

VALERIAN
Valeriana officinalis
Family: Valerianaceae

POSSIBLE USES: Valerian is a lovely flowering plant used to relieve anxiety and relax muscles. Even though it is an excellent sedative and sleep-inducing herb, it is not the source of the drug Valium as some people think. Valerian also has an antispasmodic action and is used for cramps, muscle pain, and muscle tension.

Valerian is commonly used for insomnia, tension, and nervousness. It is useful in simple cases of stress, anxiety, and nervous tension, as well as more severe cases of hysteria, nervous twitching, hyperactivity, chorea (involuntary jerky movements), heart palpitations, and tension headaches. Valerian preparations are highly regarded for insomnia. Several studies show that valerian shortens the time needed to fall asleep and improves quality of sleep. Unlike commonly used sedatives, valerian does not cause a drugged or hung-over sensation in most people.

The relaxing action of valerian also makes it useful for treatment of muscle cramps, menstrual cramps, and high blood pressure. Valerian relaxes the muscle in vein and artery walls and is especially indicated for elevated blood pressure due to stress and worry.

Valerian is approved for use by the Food and Drug Administration. It is used as a general nervine, meaning a substance that has a tonic effect on the nerves, restoring balance and relieving tension and anxiety. In the study of herbs, a nervine is classified as stimulating or sedating. Stimulating nervines are used in cases of sluggish mental activity, depression, or poor ability to concentrate, while sedating nervines are used to treat anxiety, turmoil, restlessness, and insomnia. Some herbalists consider valerian to be both stimulating and sedating, depending on the individual and the situation in which it is used. Occasionally, for example, people who use valerian to relax or improve sleep find that it worsens their complaints. Valerian is somewhat warming and stimulating, and perhaps the adverse reaction occurs in those who are already overly warm or stimulated. Valerian is best for treating depression caused by prolonged stress and nervous tension.

Valerian is mildly stimulating to the intestines, can help to dispel gas and cramps in the digestive tracts, and is weakly antimicrobial, particularly to bacteria.

POSSIBLE SIDE EFFECTS: Valerian occasionally has the opposite effect of that intended, stimulating instead of sedating. When used for insomnia, in rare cases, valerian can cause morning grogginess in some people. Reducing the dosage usually alleviates the problem. Valerian occasionally causes headaches and heart palpitations when taken in large dosages of multiple droppers full of tincture or 4 or more cups of tea per day.

PRECAUTIONS AND WARNINGS: Avoid during pregnancy. If you have thyroid disease or are typically warm-natured and tend to get hot or flushed easily, use valerian with caution or avoid altogether.

PART USED: Root, dug in the early fall

PREPARATION AND DOSAGE: Valerian root may be dried for teas or capsules or used either fresh or dried in tinctures.

Capsules: Take 2 to 3 capsules an hour before bed for insomnia or 1 or 2 capsules at a time, two to three times a day for anxiety, muscle tension, or high blood pressure.

Tincture: Take ½ to ¾ teaspoon at a time, one to three times a day for anxiety, tension, and high blood pressure. Start with a low dose and increase as needed. Take ¾ to 1 teaspoon before bed to improve insomnia.

Tea: Drink several cups of tea before bed if you don't suffer from bladder weakness. Tincture and capsules are preferred for the treatment of insomnia to prevent having a full bladder that could itself disturb sleep.

WILD YAM

Dioscorea villosa
Family: Dioscoreaceae

❧

POSSIBLE USES: *Dioscorea* is a large genus that comprises more than 600 species. Wild yam's antispasmodic and anti-inflammatory properties make it useful to treat cramps in the stomach, intestines, and bile ducts, particularly the wavelike cramping pain caused by an intestinal virus or bacteria—what we might call stomach "flu"—and colic in babies. Wild yam is also appropriate for flatulence and dysentery with cramps, especially if the conditions are caused by excess stomach acid.

POSSIBLE SIDE EFFECTS: Wild yam may aggravate or promote peptic ulcers in some people. If you experience digestive discomfort from the use of wild yam, discontinue it. If you have a history of ulcers or gastritis, use with caution. Avoid using wild yam daily, unless its use is indicated.

PRECAUTIONS AND WARNINGS: Avoid in pregnancy. Avoid in cases of peptic ulcer. Patients with metabolic disorders such as thyroid disease, diabetes, hypoglycemia, and serious infections such as hepatitis, urinary tract infections, and leukemia should avoid wild yam.

PART USED: Tubers, harvested after four or more years of growth

PREPARATION AND DOSAGE: The dried root is decocted or powdered and encapsulated. Fresh or dried root is tinctured. Wild yam may be combined with gas-relieving carminatives such as fennel or caraway seeds and soothing demulcents such as slippery elm to treat stomach pain.

Capsule: Take 2 to 4 per day.

Tincture: Take ⅛ to ½ teaspoon, three to five times a day.

Witch Hazel

Hamamelis virginiana
Family: Hamamelidaceae

❧

DESPITE ITS NAME, there is nothing to fear from this low-growing shrub, although its healing properties may seem a little like witch-craft. Actually, witch hazel may have gotten its name from its association with dowsing, which was once thought to be a form of witchcraft. Witch hazel's branches were once the wood of choice for dowsing rods, whose purpose was to locate water, or "witch" a well.

POSSIBLE USES: The bark, leaves, and twigs of witch hazel are all high in tannins, giving this plant astringent properties. Astringents are substances that can dry, tighten, and harden tissues. You may use an astringent on your skin to tighten pores and remove excess oil. A styptic pencil is a type of astringent, too, for astringents also stop discharges. The astringent tannins in witch hazel temporarily tighten and soothe aching varicose veins or reduce inflammation in cases of phlebitis (an inflammation of a vein). A cloth soaked in strong witch hazel tea reduces swelling and can relieve the pain of hemorrhoids and bruises.

Almost all pharmacies carry some type of witch hazel preparation in the form of lotions, hemorrhoidal pads, and suppositories. Besides their use topically for hemorrhoids and veins, witch hazel lotions are useful on rough, swollen gardener's or carpenter's hands.

As long as the preparation does not contain rubbing alcohol, you can use witch hazel internally to treat varicose veins, hemorrhoids, or a prolapsed uterus.

Its ability to shrink swollen tissues makes it appropriate to treat laryngitis. And a throat gargle of witch hazel, myrrh, and cloves reduces the pain of a sore throat. You can use a preparation of witch hazel and myrrh for cases of swollen and infected gums: Place a dropper full of tincture of each herb in a sip of water and use as a mouth rinse. A teaspoon of strong witch hazel tea combined with one drop each of myrrh and clove oil makes a pain- and inflammation-relieving gum rub for use in teething babies.

A cotton swab dipped in a witch hazel, goldenseal, and calendula brew and applied to the outer ear is useful in treating swimmer's ear. Swimmer's ear is associated typically with pus and moisture in the outer ear canal. Witch hazel helps dry up the secretions, while goldenseal and calendula fight infection. This same combination makes an effective vaginal douche for chronic or stubborn vaginal infections. Witch hazel combined with arnica makes an excellent topical remedy for the treatment of traumatic bruises, bumps, and sprains to both relieve pain and promote speedy healing.

Witch hazel is sometimes combined with isopropyl (rubbing) alcohol for use on external skin lesions; this form of witch hazel should not be used internally.

If you have watery stools or blood or mucus in stool chronically, your physician may suspect colitis or irritable bowel syndrome and recommend witch hazel to reduce intestinal secretions associated with these conditions. A tea made from witch hazel, chamomile, mint, and a bit of thyme can be very effective for diarrhea that accompanies an intestinal illness, or what we often call stomach "flu." For best results, an herbalist can select the right tea formula for you. If you wish to make a remedy at home, combine one tablespoon each of dried chamomile and mint and one half tablespoon of dried witch hazel and thyme. Steep in three cups of hot water.

Witch hazel is also an important botanical for controlling bleeding: It can reduce bleeding when applied topically to a wound or used internally for bleeding ulcers or bleeding gums. Of course, serious wounds require medical treatment, but witch hazel can control bleeding en route to a physician.

POSSIBLE SIDE EFFECTS: The tannins in witch hazel can produce nausea if you take it too frequently or take too large a dose at once.

PRECAUTIONS AND WARNINGS: None for the herb itself; however, do not use commercial witch hazel preparations internally if they contain isopropyl alcohol, which is a poison.

PART USED: Bark primarily, but also leaves

PREPARATION AND DOSAGE: Witch hazel is most often used topically in the form of lotions, poultices, and creams, but it is also added to tinctures and teas for internal use. Witch hazel is not recommended as a general daily beverage, but it may be consumed for cases of hemorrhoids, diarrhea, or weak, lax uterus, veins, and intestines.

Tincture: Use 10 to 40 drops two to six times daily.

Tea: Drink several cups each day, when needed. Limit use to several weeks duration.

❧ ❧ ❧

Witch Hazel Lotion

Prune witch hazel branches in the late fall or winter and shave off the bark with a sharp knife. Cut into smallish chunks with a knife or scissors, and place in a blender with enough vodka to cover the bark and blades of the blender. Chop as fine as possible, and transfer to a glass jar. Shake the mixture vigorously once a day and strain after 5 to 6 weeks. Combine 1 ounce of the witch hazel preparation with ½ ounce aloe vera gel and ½ ounce vitamin E oil and bottle.

WORMWOOD

Artemisia absinthium
Family: Compositae

POSSIBLE USES: You're not likely to forget what this herb is used for because wormwood lives up to its name. The herb has long been used to rid the body of pinworms, roundworms, and other parasites. The most common use for this bitter herb, however, is to stimulate the digestive system.

You may be familiar with the practice of taking bitters before meals to aid digestion. A bitter taste in the mouth triggers the release of bile from the gallbladder and other secretions from intestinal glands, which enable us to digest the food we eat. The promotion of bile is referred to as a cholagogue activity. People with weak digestion or insufficient stomach acid may benefit from taking wormwood preparations before meals. It's important to note, however, that if you take wormwood, you may experience diarrhea: Its secretion-stimulating qualities make the intestines empty quickly. Because wormwood also contains a substance that is toxic if consumed for a long time, wormwood is used only in small amounts for a short time.

Bitter substances have also been used to brew beer and distill alcohol. Wormwood's bitter taste comes from the substance absinthin. Absinthe, a French liqueur prepared from wormwood, is illegal because absinthol, a volatile oil the herb contains, has been found to cause nerve depression, mental impairment, and loss of reproductive function when used for a long time. Some historians believe that 19th-century painter Vincent van Gogh was addicted to absinthe. Wormwood lent its flavor and its name to vermouth. This liquor has been made since the Middle Ages, when honey and various herbs were added to wine that was beginning to sour to give it a more pleasant taste. Wormwood was one of the most common flavoring agents. The German word for wormwood is *wermuth,* which is the source of the modern word vermouth.

POSSIBLE SIDE EFFECTS: Nausea, stomach or intestinal irritation

PRECAUTIONS AND WARNINGS: Consistent use of absinthol damages the central nervous system. Don't take wormwood unless you suffer from low stomach acidity or intestinal parasites. Don't use this herb if you have excessive stomach acid, ulcers, or inflammation of the stomach.

PART USED: Leaves and flowering tops

PREPARATION AND DOSAGE: Wormwood is available fresh, tinctured, or dried for teas or for capsules.

Tea: Although they are bitter, teas are excellent for enhancing digestion as wormwood's bitter substances stimulate stomach secretions. Steep 1 teaspoon of wormwood powder in a cup of hot water for 15 minutes and drink before meals.

Capsules: Take 1 capsule before meals.

Tincture: Take 10 to 20 drops before meals.

You can buy wormwood's essential oil for use in treatment of pinworms. Pinworms and other worms become active at night, migrating to just outside the anus where the female worms lay their eggs. To kill the parasite eggs, soak a cotton ball in wormwood oil and tuck it between the buttocks at night.

YARROW

Achillea millefolium
Family: Compositae
Related Species: *A. tomentosa, A. filipendulina*

*I*N HOMER'S *ILIAD*, legendary warrior Achilles uses yarrow to treat the wounds of his fallen comrades. Indeed, constituents in yarrow make it a fine herb indeed for accelerating healing of cuts and bruises. The species name, *mille-folium,* is Latin for "a thousand leaves," referring to the herb's fine feathery foliage. Some people call it knight's milfoil, a reference to yarrow's ability to stop bleeding and promote healing of wounds.

POSSIBLE USES: Yarrow has been credited by scientists with at least minor activity on nearly every organ in the body. Early Greeks used the herb to stop hemorrhages. Yarrow was mentioned in *Gerard's Herbal* in 1597 and many herbals thereafter. Yarrow was commonly used by Native American tribes for bleeding, wounds, and infections. It is used in Ayurvedic traditions, and traditional Chinese medicine credits yarrow with the ability to affect the spleen, liver, kidney, and bladder meridians, or energy channels in the body.

Animal studies have supported the longstanding use of yarrow to cleanse wounds and control bleeding of lacerations, puncture wounds, and abrasions. Yarrow may also be used in tea or tincture form for bleeding ulcers, heavy menstrual periods, uterine hemorrhage, blood in the urine, or bleeding from the bowels. Yarrow compresses are effective for treating bleeding hemorrhoids.

Yarrow is often classified as a uterine tonic. Several studies have shown that yarrow can improve uterine tone, which may increase menstrual blood flow when it is irregular or scanty, and reduce uterine spasms, which reduces flow in cases of abnormally heavy menstrual flow. In addition to its antispasmodic activity, the herb contains salicylic acid (a compound like the active ingredient in aspirin) and volatile oil with anti-inflammatory properties, making it useful to relieve pain associated with gynecologic conditions, digestive disorders, and other conditions. Taken daily, yarrow preparations can relieve symptoms of menstrual cycle and uterine disorders such as cramps and endometriosis.

Yarrow also has antiseptic action against bacteria. The bitter constituents and fatty acids in yarrow are credited with promoting bile flow from the gallbladder, an action known as a cholagogue effect. Free-flowing bile enhances digestion and elimination and helps prevent gallstone formation. Because of these anti-inflammatory, antispasmodic, and cholagogue actions, yarrow is useful for gallbladder complaints and is considered a digestive tonic.

Yarrow has a drying effect and can be used as a decongestant. Sinus infections and coughs with sputum production may be improved by yarrow. Note that a cough with ample sputum production may be a sign of bronchitis or pneumonia and requires the attention of a physician. Yarrow's astringent action is also helpful in some cases of allergy, in which watery eyes and nasal secretions are triggered by pollen, dust, molds, and animal dander.

Yarrow also has long been used to promote sweating in cases of colds, flu, and fevers, thus helping you get over simple infections.

POSSIBLE SIDE EFFECTS: Some people may be sensitive to salicylic acid or lactone in yarrow. If you are allergic to aspirin, you may also be allergic to yarrow. The most common indicators of sensitivity are headache and nausea. No other problems are commonly reported with its use.

PRECAUTIONS AND WARNINGS: None known; however, those who are sensitive to yarrow should not use it.

PART USED: Entire herb (Flowering tops are most often used in medicines.)

PREPARATION AND DOSAGE: Fresh or dried flower tops are tinctured; dried flowers are made into teas, capsules, skin washes, and baths. You can even chew the fresh root for temporary relief of dental pain. To cleanse wounds and control bleeding, soak a cloth in strong yarrow infusion and apply it to the affected area.

Tincture: Take ¼ to ½ teaspoon, two to five times a day for treatment of upper respiratory infection, heavy menstrual bleeding, cramps, or inflammation. Start with taking it three times per day and increase or decrease as needed.

Capsules: Take 1 or 2 capsules, two to five times daily.

Yellow Dock

Rumex crispus
Family: Polygonaceae
Related Species: *Rumex acetosella* (Sheep
sorrel); *Rumex scutatus* (French sorrel)

POSSIBLE USES: Yellow dock is
commonly used as a laxative in
cases of maldigestion (diminished ability to digest foods)
and low stomach acid. Stomach
acid helps dissolve the food
you eat and break it down
into simple chemical com-
pounds the body can use.
When there is a dysfunction in
the digestive system, such as
reduced stomach acid, your
body is less able to absorb the
vitamins and minerals in foods
and eliminate waste products. *Rumex* species
stimulate intestinal secretions; these secretions
have a mild laxative effect and help eliminate
waste. They can also help bring stomach acids to
normal levels because they promote the release of
hydrochloric acid, which raises stomach acidity.
Yellow dock also promotes the flow of bile from
the liver and gallbladder, which appears to facilitate the absorption of minerals.

Like dandelion and burdock roots, yellow dock
roots and preparations are used to improve condi-

tions related to a sluggish digestive system such as liver dysfunction, acne, headaches, and constipation. Because it improves absorption of nutrients, yellow dock is also used to treat anemia and poor hair, fingernail, and skin quality. All the docks are recommended for anemia resulting from an iron deficiency because, in addition to their ability to improve the absorption of iron from the intestines, they contain a bit of iron. The docks are also high in bioflavonoids, which help strengthen capillaries.

POSSIBLE SIDE EFFECTS: Though it is unlikely that anyone would want to do so, eating several bowls full of dock salad could cause gas, cramping, diarrhea, and, if consumed to the extreme, death. Some sensitive individuals, such as those with irritable bowel syndrome, may be bothered by even small amounts of yellow dock, but a mild laxative effect is the only side effect that most people experience. Those with irritable bowels should use yellow dock cautiously, discontinuing promptly if the bowels become irritated.

PRECAUTIONS AND WARNINGS: Yellow dock contains oxalic acid, which can irritate the intestines of some people. Oxalic acid gives dock a tart, sour flavor, and it has a laxative and stimulating effect on the bowels. Oxalic acid can inflame the kidneys and intestines and should be avoided entirely by those with severe irritable bowel or kidney disease. Those with irritable digestive systems may react to even small amounts of yellow dock. Yellow dock also contains emodin, another strong laxative agent. Do not use yellow dock regularly for constipation because it can cause laxative dependence. Do not use if you have diarrhea or a history of gallbladder attacks. Do not use bitter herbs such as yellow dock or dandelion if you have pain, inflammation, or acidity in the digestive tract.

PREPARATION AND DOSAGE: The docks are short-lived perennials; if you're gathering your own, do so in the early spring or late fall. Dry the roots for teas or powder and encapsulate them. The roots, and occasionally the leaves, are also made into tinctures.

Tea: Drink several cups each day for one to two months to treat anemia.

Tincture: Take ¼ to 1 teaspoon every two to eight hours for a few days to treat constipation.

🌺 🌺 🌺
Anemia Tea

1 tsp yellow dock roots	1 Tbsp nettle leaves
1 tsp licorice root	1 Tbsp alfalfa leaves
4 cups water	

Boil yellow dock and licorice roots in water for 10 minutes. Reduce heat and simmer for 5 minutes. Add nettle and alfalfa leaves, and let stand 15 minutes more. Strain and drink 2 to 3 cups per day for one to two months.

HERB RESOURCES

HERB STARTS AND SEEDS

Seeds of Change
P.O. Box 15700
Sante Fe, NM 87506-5700

Abundant Life Seed
Foundation
P.O. Box 772
Port Townsend, WA 98368

Prairie Moon Nursery
P.O. Box 306
Westfield, WI 53964

Woodlanders, Inc.
1128 Colleton Avenue
Aiken, SC 29801

Richter's
357 Highway 47
Goodwood, ON
Canada L0C 1AO

Native Gardens
5737 Fisher Lane
Greenback, TN 37742

Missouri Wildflowers
Nursery
9814 Pleasant Hill Road
Jefferson City, MO 65109

Nature's Cathedral
1995 78th Street
Blairstown, IA 52209

Nichols' Garden Nursery
1190 North Pacific Highway
Albany, OR 97321

Thompson and Morgan, Inc.
P.O. Box 1308
Jackson, NJ 08527

Taylor's Herb Gardens
1535 Lone Oak Road
Vista, CA 92084

Logee's Greenhouses
141 North Street, Dept. IP
Danielson, CT 06239

Gardens of the Blue Ridge
P.O. Box 10
Pineola, NC 28862

BOTANICAL RETAILERS

Herb Pharm
P.O. Box 116
Williams, OR 97544

Wise Woman Herbals
1721 SE 10th Street
Portland, OR 97214

Green Terrestrial
P.O. Box 266
Milton, NY 12547

Blessed Herbs
Route 5, Box 1042
Ava, MO 65608

HERBAL ASSOCIATIONS

American Association of
Naturopathic Physicians
2366 Eastlake Avenue East,
Suite 322
Seattle, WA 98102

American Herbalist Guild
P.O. Box 1683
Soquel, CA 95073

Ontario Herbalist's
Association
P.O. Box 253, Station J
Toronto, ON
Canada M4T4Y1

American Herb Association
P.O. Box 1673
Nevada City, CA 95959

American Botanical Council
P.O. Box 201660
Austin, TX 78720-1660

Herb Research Foundation
1007 Pearl Street, Suite 200
Boulder, CO 80302

American Herbal Products
Association
4733 Bethesda Avenue,
Suite 345
Bethesda, MD 20814

International Herb Growers
and Marketers Association
1202 Allanson Road
Mundelein, IL 60060

BOTANICAL JOURNALS

HerbalGram
Mark Blumenthal, Editor
P.O. Box 201660
Austin, TX 78720-1660

The Herb Companion
Linda Ligon, Editor
201 E Fourth Street
Loveland, CO 80537

The Herb Quarterly
Linda Sparrowe, Editor
P.O. Box 689
San Anselmo, CA 94960

*American Herb Association
Newsletter*
Kathi Keville
P.O. Box 1673
Nevada City, CA 95959

*The Canadian Journal of
Herbalism*
11 Winthrop Place
Stoney Creek, ON
Canada L8G3M3

GLOSSARY

ALKALOID: Plant constituent that contains nitrogen and tends to have strong physiologic actions. Herbs that contain alkaloids include blue cohosh, comfrey, goldenseal, ma huang, motherwort, Oregon grape, and passion flower.

ALLOPATHIC: Conventional Western medicine

ALTERATIVE: Substance that gradually and favorably alters a medical condition. Alteratives also stimulate digestion and absorption of nutrients while enhancing elimination. Examples: black cohosh, burdock, echinacea, garlic, goldenseal,

ANALGESIC: Relieves pain; examples: passion flower, St. John's wort, willow bark

ANTIBIOTIC: Destroys or inhibits growth of microorganisms such as those that cause disease; examples: garlic, goldenseal, myrrh

ANTIDEPRESSANT: Elevates the mood; example, St. John's wort

ANTI-INFLAMMATORY: Reduces inflammation; examples: black cohosh, chamomile, feverfew, licorice, St. John's wort, wild yam

ANTIMICROBIAL: Destroys or inhibits the growth of disease-causing microorganisms; examples: calendula, garlic, juniper, myrrh, Oregon grape, thyme, uva ursi

ANTIOXIDANT: Prevents or delays damage from oxygen or other substances; examples: bilberry, gingko, milk thistle

ANTISEPTIC: Prevents growth of bacteria; examples: garlic, goldenseal, juniper, uva ursi, yarrow

ANTISPASMODIC: Prevents or relaxes muscle spasms; examples: black cohosh, blue cohosh, chamomile, cramp bark, dong quai, fennel, lavender, licorice, motherwort, passion flower, peppermint, skullcap, valerian, wild yam

ASTRINGENT: Dries, constricts, and shrinks inflamed or draining tissues; examples: cinnamon, goldenseal, myrrh, nettles, shepherd's purse, thyme, uva ursi, witch hazel, yarrow

BITTER: Plant with a sharp, sometimes unpalatable taste that stimulates appetite and enhances digestion; examples: burdock, dandelion, hops, Oregon grape, wormwood

CARMINATIVE: Reduces gas, bloating, and pain in the bowels; examples: chamomile, cinnamon, fennel, ginger, horseradish, hyssop, juniper, lavender, peppermint, thyme, valerian

CHOLAGOGUE: Promotes the flow of bile, which aids in fat digestion; examples: dandelion, milk thistle, Oregon grape, yellow dock

COUMARIN: Aromatic constituents of plants that can eliminate or prevent blood clots and may have antimicrobial, antispasmodic, or hormonal effects. Herbs that contain coumarin include cinnamon, dong quai, and red clover.

DEMULCENT: A soothing substance (often an oil or mucilage) that protects damaged or inflamed tissues; examples: aloe vera, comfrey, licorice, marshmallow, slippery elm, uva ursi

DIAPHORETIC: Induces sweating; examples: cayenne, garlic, ginger, peppermint, yarrow

DIURETIC: Increases urine flow; examples: burdock, dandelion, dong quai, horsetail, juniper, nettles, uva ursi, yarrow

EMMENAGOGUE: Promotes menstruation; examples: black cohosh, blue cohosh, feverfew, motherwort

EMOLLIENT: Soothes, softens, and protects skin and mucosal tissues; examples: comfrey, marshmallow

EXPECTORANT: Assists in expelling mucus from lungs and throat; examples: dong quai, hyssop, licorice, myrrh, red clover, thyme

FLAVONOID: Associated with plant pigments, flavonoids give bright yellow, orange, red, purple, and blue colors to plants. They appear to have strong physiologic effects on humans, including anti-inflammatory, antioxidant, and antimicrobial activities. They also improve the integrity of blood vessels. Herbs high in flavonoids include bilberry, chaste tree, gingko, hawthorn, milk thistle, pot marigold, and St. John's wort.

HEMOSTATIC: Arrests bleeding and promotes clotting; examples: cayenne, shepherd's purse, yarrow

LAXATIVE: Promotes bowel movements; examples: dandelion, goldenseal, licorice, Oregon grape, yellow dock

MUCILAGE: A slimy, viscous plant constituent used to soothe and hydrate tissues and reduce pain and inflamation. Comfrey roots and aloe vera leaves are high in mucilage.

NATUROPATHIC MEDICINE: A branch of modern medicine that embraces ancient natural healing traditions and merges them with modern diagnostic and scientific methods. Naturopathic medicine uses these therapies: botanical, homeopathic, hydrotherapy, traditional Chinese, Ayurvedic, massage, exercise, nutrition, emotional, and spiritual. It may employ laboratory tests, X rays, spinal manipulation, surgery, and pharmaceuticals associated with traditional Western medicine.

NATUROPATHIC PHYSICIAN: A licensed primary care physician who has completed doctoral level training in naturopathic medicine and specializes in natural therapies.

NERVINE: Calms tension and nourishes the nervous system; examples: skullcap, valerian

ORGANIC ACIDS: Weak acids that occur commonly in plants, particularly fruits; the citric acid in lemons is an organic acid. These acids have an irritant, laxative effect on the bowels. Yellow dock is high in laxative organic acids.

PHYTOSTEROL: Plant steroids. While most phytosterols are not identical to human steroids, they do appear to affect our hormones. Many plants high in steroids are used for menopausal complaints, menstrual irregularities, infertility, and muscle building. Phytosterols may be categorized further as steroidal saponins or steroidal alkaloids.

RESIN: A sticky, thick fluid in the tissues of some plants. Resins act as stimulants, expectorants, and antimicrobials and are used in skin, lung, and kidney remedies. Ginger, juniper, myrrh, and red clover are examples of plants high in resins.

RUBEFACIENT: Increases blood flow at the skin surface, causing reddening; examples: cayenne, ginger, horseradish

SAPONIN: Plant constituents usually found bound to a sugar molecule. Structurally, saponins are similar to steroids, and, indeed, many plants high in saponins have a hormone-like activity in the body. Herbs that contain saponins include blue cohosh, ginger, and licorice.

SEDATIVE: Quiets the nervous system and promotes sleep; examples: black cohosh, hops, lavender, passion flower, skullcap, valerian

STIMULANT: Increases energy and circulation; examples: cayenne, cinnamon, ginger, horseradish

Succus: Juice expressed for medicinal purposes and stabilized with a low concentration of alcohol

Synergist: Enhances the action of a medicinal substance.

Tannin: A plant constituent that dries and tightens skin and internal tissues. Tannins are most prominent in plant leaves and bark, such as witch hazel bark. They are used topically on wounds to promote drying and scabbing over and internally to heal ulcers.

Tonic: Improves organ or tissue function; examples: ginseng, goldenseal, hawthorn, nettles

Topical: Intended for direct application to the skin

Volatile Oils or Essential Oils: The strong aroma-producing substances in a plant. They are "volatile" because they are unstable compounds given off freely into the atmosphere. Plants produce volatile oils to attract pollinators, so the oils are most abundant usually when the plant is flowering. Medicinal herbs high in volatile oils include chamomile, peppermint, thyme, wormwood, and valerian.

Vulnerary: Encourages healing of wounds; examples: aloe vera, calendula, comfrey, marshmallow, myrrh, oats, St. John's wort

INDEX

Flu. *See also* Stomach flu.
  echinacea for, 115, 117
  garlic for, 125, 128
  horseradish for, 153
  licorice for, 165
  ma huang for, 170
  Oregon grape for, 188
  slippery elm for, 216
  yarrow for, 237
Food poisoning, 97–98

G
Gallbladder, 194, 237, 241
Gallstones, 107, 194
Garlic, 45, 47, 50, 55, 124–128
Gas
  chamomile for, 91
  cinnamon for, 97
  dandelion for, 107
  fennel for, 118
  ginger for, 130
  goldenseal for, 143
  juniper for, 158
  lavender for, 160
  lemon balm for, 163
  peppermint for, 192
  sage for, 201
  valerian for, 224
  wild yam for, 226
  from yellow dock, 240
Gastritis, 68, 226
Genital inflammation, 83
Ginger, 40, 47, 49, 52, 55, 58,
    129–132, 176
Gingivitis, 178
Ginkgo, 40, 133–136
Ginseng, 40, 137–141
Glands, swollen, 55
Gobo root. *See* Burdock.
Goldenseal, 40, 51, 52, 91, 142–146,
    229
Gout, 158, 180–181
Greek medicine, 12–15
Gums, bleeding or infected, 82, 99,
    143, 178, 229, 230

H
Hair, herbs for, 240
Harvesting herbs, 32–34
Hawthorn, 40, 147–149
Hay fever, 170, 219
Headaches
  black cohosh and, 74
  compresses for, 55

Headaches (*continued*)
  dandelion for, 107
  feverfew for, 120–121, 123
  from ginkgo, 135, 136
  from hops, 151
  lavender for, 160
  motherwort for, 177
  from peppermint, 193
  peppermint for, 193
  from valerian, 225
  valerian for, 223
  from yarrow, 237
  yellow dock for, 240
Heartburn, 68, 80, 194
Heart palpitations, 148, 170, 176,
    177, 223, 225
Heart rate, rapid, 88, 176
Hemorrhages, 170, 211
Hemorrhoids, 68, 83, 205, 228, 229,
    231, 236
Hepatitis, 188, 214, 227
Herbalist, consulting, 28–29
Herpes, 87, 125, 163, 165
Hiatal hernia, 194
High blood pressure
  black cohosh for, 74
  cayenne pepper for, 86
  cinnamon and, 97, 98
  dandelion for, 105
  dong quai and, 112, 113
  ginseng and, 140, 141
  hawthorn for, 148
  horsetail and, 156
  lemon balm for, 163
  licorice and, 93, 167
  ma huang and, 171
  motherwort for, 177
  passion flower for, 190
  valerian for, 223–224, 225
Hoarseness, 216
Hookworms, 219
Hops, 40, 58, 150–151
Horehound, 40
Hormone balance, 64, 80, 165
Horseradish, 45, 152–154
Horsetail, 40, 155–156
Hyperactivity, 223
Hypertension. *See* High blood
    pressure.
Hypoglycemia, 177,
    227
Hyssop, 40